BASIC
ENGLISH
CONVERSATION
IN THE DENTAL CLINIC

베이직 통합치과영어

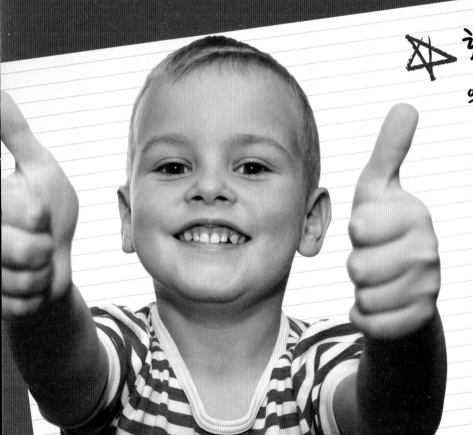

환자의 입장
의료인 입장에서의
영어 의미 표현

천세희 지음

KOONJA

베이직 통합 치과영어

Basic English Conversation in the Dental Clinic

첫째판 1쇄 인쇄 | 2015년 8월 20일
첫째판 1쇄 발행 | 2015년 8월 25일
첫째판 2쇄 발행 | 2019년 1월 18일

지 은 이 천세희
발 행 인 장주연
출 판 기 획 군자기획부
편집디자인 군자편집부
표지디자인 군자표지부
발 행 처 군자출판사(주)
　　　　 등록 제4-139호(1991. 6. 24)
　　　　 본사 (10881) **파주출판단지** 경기도 파주시 회동길 338(서패동 474-1)
　　　　 전화 (031) 943-1888 　 팩스 (031) 955-9545
　　　　 홈페이지 | www.koonja.co.kr

ISBN 978-89-6278-238-7

정가 20,000원

지은이 **천세희**

Certification of Completion - Sydney Practical English & Communication College.

Statement of Attainment in Advanced English

-New South Wales Technical and Further Education Commission Australia.

치과병원 치과위생사 근무

어학원 영어강사 근무

영어학부 실용영어 전공

(현) 동의대학교 치위생학과 조교수

(현) 대한치과위생사협회 국제이사

보건학 박사 졸업

Preface

치과위생사이면서 영어전공자가 치과생활영어의 필요성에 대한 동기유발을 심어주기를 원했습니다. 그러나 기존의 치과생활영어는 저의 수업방식에 맞는 책이 없었기에 어떻게 하면 치위생(학)과 학생들에게 흥미롭고 재미있게 치과생활영어를 가르칠 수 있을지... 고민을 하다가 어휘뿐만 아니라 회화, 듣기, 읽기, 그리고 영작까지 잘 할 수 있는 통합적인 영어 커리큘럼이 필요하다는 생각을 하였습니다. 문법에 의존하고 해석에만 치우치는 그런 생활영어가 아니라 일반적인 의료어휘, 읽기, 듣기, 말하기, 또한 자기소개서와 이력서를 작성하는 영작까지 모든 영역을 이 책 한권에 담아보았습니다.

의료전문가가 사용하는 의학용어는 일반적인 외국인환자는 잘 알지 못합니다. 의학전문용어는 의료인이기 때문에 당연히 숙지해야 하고 외국인환자와 의사소통할 때는 영어단어로 알기 쉽게 설명하여야 합니다. 의학전문용어를 영어로 생각하고 외국인환자에게 설명하다보면 잘 못 알아 듣거나 의사소통이 잘 안되어 난처하기도 합니다.

이 책은 각각의 영역별로 구성되어져 있으며 중간 중간에 연습문제와 액티비티로 본인의 영어실력을 체크할 수 있도록 했습니다. 역할극을 통하여 영어대본을 만들었으며 각 상황을 설정하여 프리젠테이션하는 것 또한 영어와 한걸음 더 친숙할 수 있도록 했습니다.

또한 이 책에서는 한글해석을 달지 않았습니다. 영어와 한글을 나란히 배열하면 대부분 사람들은 영어보다 한글 쪽으로 눈이 먼저 갑니다. 따라서 영어를 한번 읽어보고 모르는 단어는 스스로 찾아서 해석하고 구음함으로서 자연스럽게 영어공부를 하고자 의도한 것입니다.

주위사람들이 저에게 묻습니다. 어떻게 하면 영어를 잘 할 수 있냐고, 전 매일 조금씩 그리고 영어를 가르치면서 배우기도 하고, 항상 영어사전을 이용하여 참고문장 및 단어의 부연설명까지 참고를 합니다. 조금씩 노력하다보면 영어와 친숙하게 될 것이며 소리 내어 읽어보는 것도 큰 도움이

된다고 생각합니다. 영어 울렁증이나 영어와 담을 쌓으신 분에게 팁이 될지 모르겠지만 영어에 대한 갈망을 항상 마음속에 품고 있으면 상당히 발전할 수 있는 가능성이 있다고 생각합니다.

글로벌시대에 의료관광, 의료인 해외진출 등... 영어는 이젠 선택이 아니라 필수의 시대가 되었습니다. 이 책이 치과위생사들의 경쟁력을 키울 수 있고 세계로 진출할 수 있는, 내공있는 학계로 거듭 태어날 수 있는 밑거름이 되었으면 합니다.
이 책 한 권으로 생활영어를 마스터 할 수는 없겠지만 조금이나마 기억에 남고 영어와 친해질 수 있었으면 합니다. 또한 가장 중요한 것은 한 차원 높은 치과위생사가 되고 싶다면 영어와 사이좋게 손잡고 함께 동반할 수 있기를 기원해봅니다.

이 책에 관한 조언과 항상 긍정의 에너지를 주시는 제 은사님이신 권현숙 교수님, 힘들 때 찾아뵙고 오면 마음의 평정을 찾게 해주시는 정성화 지도교수님, 제 주위에 도움주신 모든 분들에게 감사의 표현과 이 책을 펴는데 친근하게 도움을 주신 군자출판사 관계자 여러분들에게 감사의 마음을 전합니다.

2015. 8월 저자

Contents

4. DIALOGUE

5. NARRATIVE

6. WRITING

Pronunciation

L and **R**	L	walk, light, long, lane, fly
	R	work, right, wrong, rain, fry
F and **P**	F	face, fan, fast, fool, coffee
	P	pace, pan, past, pool, copy
B and **V**	B	berry, boat, base, bent, ban
	V	very, vote, vase, vent, van

Tongue Twisters

Peter Piper picked a peck of pickled peppers.
Shy Shelly says she shall sew sheets.
Which witch wished which wicked wish?
A big clack bear sat on a big black bug.
Red lolly, yellow lolly, red lolly, yellow lolly

1

Vocabulary

Intro

국어와 마찬가지로 영어에서도 전문 의학용어와 외국인이 사용하는 영어의학용어 사용이 다르다. Part 1에서는 어휘력 중심으로 병원에서 사용하는 용어, 질병에 관련된 용어 및 기타 건강에 관련된 일반적인 용어와 문장으로 구성되어져 있다. 의료전문가들이 알고 있는 전문 의학용어들 뿐만 아니라 평소에 외국인 환자들이 사용하고 있는 영어단어로 정리돼 있으며 쉽게 접할 수 있는 영어 단어의 의미를 한 번 더 알아보고, 치과위생사들 또한 기본적인 영어의 의미를 숙지할 필요가 있다. 기본적인 영어의미를 숙지한 다음 연습문제를 통하여 어휘력 향상을 체크해 보자.

01

병원에서
사용하는 단어 I

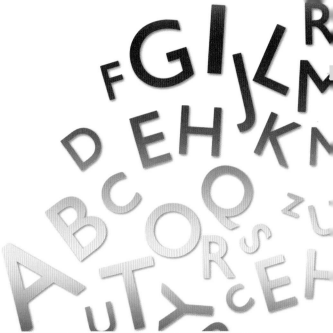

01. acupuncture	The treatment of a person's illness or pain by sticking small needles into their body at certain places. Acupuncture has also been shown to relieve pain after dental procedures.
02. antibody	Substances which a person's or an animal's body produces n their blood in order to destroy substances which carry disease. Antibodies from the mother's milk line the baby's intestine and prevent infection.
03. artificial	Made by human skill, produced by humans. An artificial heart keeps patients alive until they receive a heart transplant.

04. antibiotics	Medical drugs used to kill bacteria and treat infections.
	Antibiotics remain our most effective weapon against disease causing bacteria.
05. autopsy	An examination of a dead body by a doctor who cuts it open in order to try to discover the cause of death.
	A medical autopsy is another tool used by the criminal.
06. black out	To lose consciousness or memory temporarily.
	The driver had probably blacked out at the wheel.
07. blood donation	The acting giving to his or her blood to be used for transfusion.
	There is no maximum age limit for blood donation as long as the donor is healthy.
08. bruise	An injury which appears as a purple mark on your body, although the skin is not broken.
	Thankfully the only injuries. I've had a few bruises and a fat lip.
	His arms and chest were covered in bruise.
09. bump	A minor injury or swelling that you get if you bump into something or if something hits you.
	She bumped into a server, knocking the food from the tray onto other customers.
	Tim had a bump on his head.

10. burn

If you burn part of your body, burn yourself, or are burnt, you are injured by fire or by something very hot.

The child was badly burnt in the fire.

11. call in sick

If you call in sick, you telephone the place where you work to tell them you will not be coming to work cause you are ill.

He is out sick today. He called in sick today.

12. care for

To take care of and be responsible for somebody who is cry young, old or sick, etc.

The children are being care for by a relative.

13. carry out

To perform or cause to be implemented.

The hospital is carrying out tests to find what's wrong with her kidney.

14. cavity

A cavity is a hole in a tooth, caused by decay.

She recently developed a cavity in one of her lower back teeth.

15. checkup

A check-up is a medical examination by your doctor or dentist to make sure that there is nothing wrong with your health.

She goes to her dentist for regular check-ups.

16. choke

When you choke or when something chokes you, you cannot breathe properly or get enough air into your lungs.

Children can choke on peanuts.

Six people choked to death on the fumes.

The pictures of starving children choked me up.

17. come down with

To get an illness, often not a very serious one.

It says, women living in slums are also more likely to come down with HIV/AIDS than their rural counterparts.

18. conduct

When you conduct an activity or task, you organize it and carry it out.

We conduct emission tests to detect whether the products we use emit harmful gasses.

19. conscious

If you are conscious of something, you notice it or realize that it is happening.

Today, many more people have become conscious of what is happening to their waste.

20. contagious

A disease that is contagious can be caught by touching people or things that are infected with it.

Am I contagious? Do I need to be isolated?

21. contract

If you contract a serious illness, you become ill with it.

He seems to have contracted malaria through an insect bite.

22. decease

A more formal word for death.

The house will be yours after your mother's decease.

23. dental braces

A device used in orthodontics to align teeth and their position with regard to a person's bite.

When I was a teenager, I had to wear dental braces for my crooked teeth.

24. diagnose

If someone or something is diagnosed as having a particular illness or problem, their illness or problem is identified.

My aunt and my best friend's mom were recently diagnosed with breast cancer.

25. disabled

Someone who is disabled has an illness, injury, or condition that tends to restrict the way that they can live their life, especially by making it difficult for them to move about.

The accident left him severely disabled.

26. disease

A disease is an illness which affects people, animals, or plants, for example one which is caused by bacteria or infection.

One of the symptoms of the disease is a very high temperature.

27. dose

A dose of medicine or a drug is a measured amount of it which is intended to be taken at one time.

The label says you should take one dose three times a day.

28. euthanasia

Euthanasia is the practice of killing someone who is very ill and will never get better in order to end their suffering, usually done at their request or with their consent.

Euthanasia is still illegal in most countries.

29. emergency

An emergency is an unexpected and difficult or dangerous situation, especially an accident, which happens suddenly and which requires quick action to deal with it.

He will be absent today because of a family emergency.

30. examine

If a doctor examines you, he or she looks at your body, feels it, or does simple tests in order to check how healthy you are.

A doctor examined my back and suggested. I have surgery.

31. experiment

An experiment is a scientific test which is done in order to discover what happens to something in particular conditions.

Experiments on animals should be banned.

32. faint

If you faint, you lose consciousness for a short time, especially because you are hungry, or because of pain, heat, or shock. Someone who is faint feels weak and unsteady as if they are about to lose consciousness.

She fainted in the scorching sunlight.

I felt faint with hunger.

33. fatal

A fatal accident or illness causes someone's death.

She suffered a fatal injury to her head.

There were a few fatal flaws in the representative's argument.

34. filling

A filling is a small amount of metal or plastic that a dentist puts in a hole in a tooth to prevent further decay.

Gold fillings are durable enough to withstand chewing forces.

My filling has fallen out.

35. first aid

First aid is simple medical treatment given as soon as possible to a person who is injured or who suddenly becomes ill.

Did you learn any first aid at school?

36. fit

Someone who is fit is healthy and physically strong.

I jog to keep fit.

37. fracture

A fracture is a slight crack or break in something, especially a bone.

He sustained multiple fractures in a motorcycle accident.

38. frostbite

Frostbite is a condition in which parts of your body, such as your fingers or toes, become seriously damaged as a result of being very cold.

I was in extreme pain from the frostbite and my other injuries.

EXERCISE 1

A 주어진 단어를 이용하여 문장을 완성하시오.

1. cavity ( )

2. diagnose ( )

3. conscious ( )

B 빈칸에 들어갈 알맞은 것을 〈보기〉에서 고르시오.

〈보기〉 emergency   bruise   unconscious   choked   frostbitten   fatal

1. You are suppose to ice a _____ when you first get it.

2. The average fever of 108 is considered to be _____ and may cause brain damage.

3. Charlie remained _____ and in critical condition.

4. I _____ up a little bit leaving my house today.

밑줄 친 부분과 뜻이 가장 가까운 것을 고르시오.

1. My dentists said I have four <u>cavities</u> that need to be filled.

   (a) teeth   (b) drills   (c) gums   (d) tooth decay   (e) molars

2. <u>Contagious</u> diseases that pose a health risk to people have always existed.

   (a) severe   (b) various   (c) unknown   (d) precarious   (e) infectious

3. A boy with severe burns has gone through an <u>artificial</u> skin transplant.

   (a) ubiquitous   (b) auxiliary   (c) blatant   (d) plentiful   (e) man-made

4. There are simple home chores to stay <u>fit</u>; such as sweeping the porch, pulling weeds by hand, and dusting the furnitures.

   (a) calm   (b) healthy   (c) organized   (d) handsome   (e) ridiculous

02

병원에서
사용하는 단어 Ⅱ

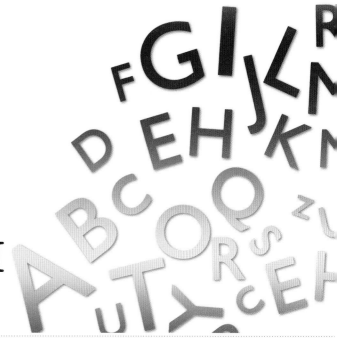

01. germ	A germ is a very small organism that causes disease.
	Pneumonia is a lung infection that can be caused by a number of germs.
	Rats and flies have to be exterminated because they spread germs.
02. get well	To improve in health. "He got well fast".
	I'm very glad you got well so quickly.
03. handicapped	Someone who is handicapped has a physical or mental disability that prevents them living a totally normal life.
	His example has encouraged both handicapped and healthy people to attempt the impossible.
04. hangover	If someone wakes up with a hangover, they feel sick and have a headache because they have drunk a lot of alcohol the night before.
	It seems like that he has a hangover this morning.

05. health insurance	Insurance against expenses incurred through illness of the insured.
	All citizens are covered by national health insurance.
06. hospitalize	If someone is hospitalized, they are sent or admitted to hospital.
	My wife has been hospitalized after the car accident.
07. immunization	The fact or process of becoming immune, as against a disease.
	Could you give me a hepatitis immunization?
08. intensive care	If someone is in intensive care, they are being given extremely thorough care in a hospital because they are very ill or very badly injured.
	It is not possible for all patients to receive intensive care.
09. infection	An infection is a disease caused by germs or bacteria to infect people, animals, or plants means to cause them to have a disease or illness.
	Please bandage the wound to reduce the risk of infection.
	All of the children here are infected with an unknown virus.

10. inflammation

An inflammation is a painful redness or swelling of a part of your body that results from an infection, injury, or illness.

This injection will reduce pain and inflammation.

11. injection

If you have an injection, a doctor or nurse puts a medicine into your body using a device with a needle called a syringe.

This drug can be given by injection.

The doctor gave me a shot of morphine.

12. injured

An injured person or animal has physical damage to part of their body, usually as a result of an accident or fighting.

He was told to stay in bed to rest his injured leg.

13. injury

An injury is damage done to a person's or an animal's body

Some passengers sustained serious injuries in the train crash.

14. IV (intravenous)

Intravenous foods or drugs are given to sick people through their veins, rather than their mouths.

An IV drip hangs by her bed.

15. medication

Medication is medicine that is used to treat and cure illness.

Are you taking any medication?

He is currently on medication for his kidneys.

16. mental

Mental means relating to the state or the health of a person's mind.

As time passed, her physical and mental health got worse.

17. obesity

The condition of being very fat or overweight.

Obesity is defined as having an excessive amount of body fat.

18. ointment

An ointment is a smooth thick substance that is put on sore skin or a wound to help it heal.

You need to apply some ointment.

19. operation

When a patient has an operation, a surgeon cuts open their body in order to remove, replace, or repair a diseased or damaged part.

He's got to have an operation on his shoulder.

Are they going to operate on him?

20. organ

An organ is a part of your body that has a particular purpose or function, for example your heart or lungs.

You can save the lives of many people if you register yourself as an organ donor.

21. over-the-counter drugs	A drug that is sold without a prescription.
	There are some teens and young adults abusing over-the-counter drugs.
22. paralyze	Cause (a person or part of the body) to become partly or wholly incapable of movement.
	He fell from a horse and was paralyzed down one side of his body.
23. pass away	People say pass away to avoid saying die.
	I was greatly astonished to hear his passing away.
24. pass out	To become unconscious, faint.
	She was hit on the head and passed out.
	I nearly fainted in the heat.
25. pediatrician	A pediatrician is a doctor who specializes in treating sick children.
	He asked the pediatrician a question about his son's health.
	Ms. Smith specializes in pediatrics.
26. perish	If people or animals perish, they die as a result of very harsh conditions or as the result of an accident.
	Three hundred people perished in the earthquake.

27. pharmacy

A pharmacy is a shop or a department in a shop where medicines are sold or given out.

Is there an all-night pharmacy near here?

28. physical

Physical qualities, actions, or things are connected with a person's body, rather than with their mind.

She is obsessed with physical appearance.

29. physician

In formal American English or old-fashioned British English, a physician is a doctor.

I am a nurse practitioner and my husband is a physician.

30. pill

Pills are small solid round masses of medicine or vitamins that you swallow without chewing.

My mother takes three or four of these pills a day.

31. plastic surgery

Plastic surgery is the practice of performing operations to repair or replace skin which has been damaged, or to improve people's appearance.

She had plastic surgery on her nose.

32. prescribe

If a doctor prescribes medicine or treatment for you, he or she tells you what medicine or treatment to have.

The medicine is often prescribed for depression.

33. pulse

Your pulse is the regular beating of blood through your body, which you can feel when you touch particular parts of your body, especially your wrist.

Her pulse is very weak.

34. recover

When you recover from an illness or an injury, you become well again.

It took her a long time to recover from her operation. Police recovered only a few stolen items.

35. rehabilitate

To rehabilitate someone who has a drug or alcohol problem means to help them stop using drugs or alcohol.

There is a special facility for rehabilitating alcoholics.

36. remedy

If you remedy something that is wrong or harmful, you correct it or improve it.

We must act quickly to remedy this situation.

37. saliva

Saliva is the watery liquid that forms in your mouth and helps you to chew and digest food.

Saliva has an important role in preventing tooth decay.

38. shape

The particular condition or state of someone or something.

"How are you doing?" "I'm in great shape, thanks."

39. side effect

The side effects of a drug are the effects, usually bad ones, that the drug has on you in addition to its function of curing illness or pain.

Does this drug have any side effects?

40. spit

If someone spits, they force an amount of liquid out of their mouth, often to show hatred or contempt.

Spit is the watery liquid produced in your mouth.

You usually use spit to refer to an amount of it that has been forced out of someone's mouth.

He spat the meat out in disgust.

The teacher spits a lot.

She washed off her baby's face covered with his spit.

41. sprain

If you sprain a joint such as your ankle or wrist, you accidentally damage it by twisting it or bending it violently.

While your strain or sprain heels, take good care of your injury by resting the injured part of your body.

42. stethoscope

A stethoscope is an instrument that a doctor uses to listen to your heart and breathing.

Will you hand me the stethoscope?

43. suffer

If you suffer from an illness or from some other bad condition, you are badly affected by it.

She's been suffering from cancer for several years.

44. suffocate

If someone suffocates or is suffocated, they die because there is no air for them to breathe.

The police report said that the victims had suffocated in the fumes.

45. surgeon

A surgeon is a doctor who is specially trained to perform surgery.

The surgeon passes the laparoscope through an incision in your abdomen.

46. surgery

Surgery is medical treatment in which someone's body is cut open so that a doctor can repair, remove, or replace a diseased or damaged part.

The patient had brain surgery.

47. swell (up)

If the amount or size of something swells or if something swells it, it becomes larger than it was before.

His twisted ankle began to swell.

48. therapy

Therapy is the treatment of someone with mental or physical illness without the use of drugs or operations.

He does twice the prescribed amount of physical therapy.

49. tooth decay

If you have tooth decay, one or more of your teeth has become decayed.

Tooth decay is one of the most common health complaints in the world.

50. transfusion

An act of transfusing donated blood, blood products, or other fluid into the circulatory system of a person or animal.

A blood transfusion is needed to save her life.

51. transmit

If one person or animal transmits a disease to another, they have the disease and cause the other person or animal to have it.

Many diseases are transmitted through contaminated water.

52. transplant

A transplant is a medical operation in which a part of a person's body is replaced because it is diseased.

He is waiting for a kidney transplant.

53. treatment

Treatment is medical attention given to a sick or injured person or animal.

The victims were given emergency treatment by paramedics.

He is being treated for cancer.

54. vaccine

A vaccine is a substance containing a harmless form of the germs that cause a particular disease.

It is given to people, usually by injection, to prevent them getting that disease.

This vaccine protects people against flu viruses.

55. ward

A ward is a room in a hospital which has beds for many people, often people who need similar treatment. To prevent somebody/something dangerous or unpleasant from affecting or harming you.

There are many patients in the ward.

Take this bug repellent to ward off the mosquitos.

56. wound

A wound is damage to part of your body, especially a cut or a hole in your flesh, which is caused by a gun, knife, or other weapon.

It took several weeks for his wounds to heal.

EXERCISE 2

 주어진 단어를 이용하여 문장을 완성하시오.

1. hangover ( )

2. infection ( )

3. health insurance ( )

B 빈칸에 들어갈 알맞은 것을 〈보기〉에서 고르시오.

〈보기〉 prescription   immunization   organs   cured   paralyzed

1. James is _____ as the result of an all-terrain vehicle accident.

2. Celebration seeking a botox job will have to get a doctor's _____ before getting the wrinkle-busting jab.

3. Fatty foods that harden arteries may also harm vital _____.

4. Ulcers in 16 of 29 people who received the drug have been _____ completely.

밑줄 친 부분과 뜻이 가장 가까운 것을 고르시오.

1. Two people died after an adverse reaction to a malaria <u>injection</u>.

   (a) treatment   (b) transfusion   (c) hangover   (d) injury   (e) shot

2. Enzymes in the <u>saliva</u> digest the sugars in milks and juices.

   (a) ointment   (b) spit   (c) medication   (d) transplant   (e) tears

3. My son broke his arm and had to wear a <u>cast</u> from his wrist to elbow.

   (a) wig   (b) glove   (c) plaster   (d) sling   (e) hood

4. This drug provides a new <u>therapy</u> for HIV patients with limited treatment.

   (a) remedy   (b) congestion   (c) antibody   (d) pulse   (e) rehab

03

질병 및 증상을
나타내는 단어

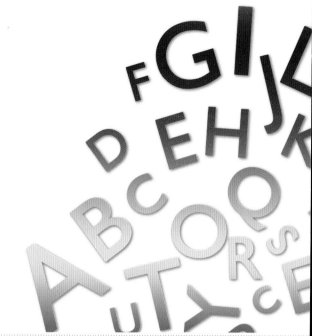

---

01. acute

An acute illness is one that becomes severe very quickly but does not last very long.

We can prevent chronic and acute respiratory infections through the use of better fuels.

02. Alzheimer's

Alzheimer's disease is a condition in which a person's brain gradually stops working properly.

At the end stages of the disease, Alzheimer's patients are generally bedridden and unable to communicate.

03. amnesia

If someone is suffering from amnesia, they have lost their memory.

She suffered periods of amnesia in her later life.

04. anemia

Anemia is a medical condition in which there are too few red cells in your blood, causing you to feel tired and look pale.

Anemia may cause tiredness and pallor.

05. anorexia

Anorexia or anorexia nervosa is an illness in which a person has an overwhelming fear of becoming fat, and so refuses to eat enough and becomes thinner and thinner.

Eating disorders such as anorexia are on the rise.

06. arthritis

Arthritis is a medical condition in which the joints in someone's body are swollen and painful.

Some children with arthritis have poor appetites.

07. asthma

Asthma is a lung condition which causes difficulty in breathing.

A very severe asthma attack can lead to respiratory arrest and death.

08. bird flu

Also called avian flu a form of influenza occurring in poultry mainly in Japan, China and Southeast Asia, caused by a virus capable of spreading to humans.

Bird flu viruses infect bird including chickens and wild bird.

09. blister

A blister is a painful swelling on the surface of your skin. Blisters contain a clear liquid and are usually caused by heat or by something repeatedly rubbing your skin.

I burnt my feet over the weekend, and they're starting to blister.

They went out in the blistering heat.

10. bloodshot

If your eyes are bloodshot, the parts that are usually white are red or pink.

Her eyes were bloodshot from lack of sleep.

11. bloody nose

A nose that is bleeding internally.

Can you tell me how to stop a bloody nose?

12. bulimia

Bulimia or bulimia nervosa is an illness in which a person has a very great fear of becoming fat, and so they make themselves vomit after eating.

The Princess of Wales was widely reported to have suffered from bulimia throughout her 20s.

13. cancer

Cancer is a serious disease in which cells in a person's body increase rapidly in an uncontrolled way, producing abnormal growths.

He died of liver cancer last year.

14. chicken pox

Chicken pox is a disease which gives you a high temperature and red spots that itch.

Chicken pox is a very common disease among children.

15. cholera

Cholera is a serious disease that often kills people.

It is caused by drinking infected water or by eating infected food.

Cholera is a bacterial disease which affects the intestinal tract.

16. chronic

A chronic illness or disability lasts for a very long time.

He suffered from chronic depression.

17. cold

If you have a cold, you have a mild, very common illness which makes you sneeze a lot and gives you a sore throat or a cough.

She has caught a cold.

My feet are so cold.

It's freezing cold today.

18. constipation

Constipation is a medical condition which causes people to have difficulty getting rid of solid waste from their body.

Not only humans but pets can suffer from constipation.

You need to consume more fiber so you won't get constipated.

19. cough	When you cough, you force air out of your throat with a sudden, harsh noise.
	Please, cover your mouth when you cough or sneeze.
20. diabetes	Diabetes is a medical condition in which someone has too much sugar in their blood.
	Diabetes affects an estimated 17 million Americans, and the number is increasing each year.
21. diarrhea	If someone has diarrhoea, a lot of liquid faeces comes out of their body because they are ill.
	Orlistat blocks fat absorption, but can result in side effects like gas and diarrhea.
22. dizzy	If you feel dizzy, you feel that you are losing your balance and are about to fall.
	I get easily short of breath and dizzy.
23. drowsy	If you feel drowsy, you feel sleepy and cannot think clearly.
	I'm taking some cold medicine, which makes me drowsy.
24. earache	Earache is a pain in the inside part of your ear.
	I have an earache.

25. fever	If you have a fever when you are ill, your body temperature is higher than usual and your heart beats faster.
	He's got a headache and a slight fever.
	The Japanese fever hit Asia in the 1990s.
26. heart attack	If someone has a heart attack, their heart begins to beat very irregularly or stops completely.
	John had a heart attack three years ago.
27. high blood pressure	Elevation of the arterial blood pressure or a condition resulting from it.
	When you have high blood pressure, the blood pressure in the arteries is elevated.
28. insomnia	Someone who suffers from insomnia finds it difficult to sleep.
	Holly suffered from insomnia for months after her mother's death.
29. itchy	If a part of your body or something you are wearing is itchy, you have an unpleasant feeling on your skin that makes you want to scratch.
	The sweater made me feel itchy all over.
	I can't wear wool because it makes me itch.
	I have an itch a visit to Japan.
	I'm itching for a visit to Japan.

30. leprosy	Leprosy is an infectious disease that damages people's flesh.
	Leprosy has been a dreaded condition since the beginning of human history.
31. leukemia	A type of cancer of the blood or bone marrow characterized by an abnormal increase of immature white blood cells called "blasts".
	Babies who are breast-feed have a lower risk of developing leukemia.
32. mad cow disease	Mad cow disease is a disease which affects the nervous system of cattle and causes death.
	Demand for pork increased following the outbreak of mad cow disease.
33. measles	Measles is an infectious illness that gives you a high temperature and red spots on your skin.
	Measles is best known for its typical skin rash.
34. motion sickness	The state or condition of being dizzy or nauseous from riding in a moving vehicle.
	Ginger may help prevent motion sickness.
35. nauseous	If you feel nauseous, you feel as if you want to vomit.
	I felt nauseous after eating sashimi.
	Just the thought of that medicine makes me queasy.

36. pale	If something is pale, it is very light in colour or almost white.
	You're looking pale.
37. pneumonia	Pneumonia is a serious disease which affects your lungs and makes it difficult for you to breathe.
	The cold worsened and turned into pneumonia.
38. runny nose	Persistent watery mucus discharge from the nose.
	I've got a runny nose today.
39. sneeze	When you sneeze, you suddenly take in your breath and then blow it down your nose noisily without being able to stop yourself, for example because you have a cold.
	Cats make me sneeze I guess I'm allergic to the fur.
40. snore	When someone who is asleep snores, they make a loud noise each time they breathe.
	He snores so loudly. It keeps me awake at night.
	I couldn't put up with his terrible snore.
41. sore	If part of your body is sore, it causes you pain and discomfort.
	All the dust particles made my eyes sore.
	Is this an eyesore to you?

42. strain

Strain is an injury to a muscle in your body, caused by using the muscle too much or twisting it.

Your bones are so weak that a sudden strain can cause a fracture.

Excess weight puts a lot of strain on your heart.

A new, more dangerous strain of the virus has been found.

43. stroke

If someone has a stroke, a blood vessel in their brain bursts or becomes blocked, which may kill them or make them unable to move one side of their body.

Stroke is a medical emergency, and prompt treatment of a stroke is crucial.

44. stuffy

Affected with a sensation of obstruction in the respiratory passages.

These pills may ease your stuffy nose.

45. symptom

A symptom of an illness is something wrong with your body or mind that is a sign of the illness.

She's started to develop the symptoms of HIV.

46. terminal

A terminal illness or disease causes death, often slowly and cannot be cured.

She was diagnosed with terminal lung cancer.

47. throw up

To bring food you have eaten back out of your mouth.

I feel like throwing up.

He vomitted this morning.

A 주어진 단어를 이용하여 문장을 완성하시오.

1. amnesia ( )

2. sore ( )

3. chronic ( )

B 빈칸에 들어갈 알맞은 것을 〈보기〉에서 고르시오.

〈보기〉 diabetes   amnesia   asthma   arthritis   leukemia

1. The senator died from complications of _____ thursday morning.

2. Patients suffering from _____ may have worse health-related quality of life than those with other chronic conditions.

3. Patients with _____ have a much higher rate of hypertension.

4. _____ medicines are normally taken using an inhaler.

밑줄 친 부분과 뜻이 가장 가까운 것을 고르시오.

1. I felt <u>nauseous</u> again and ended up vomiting.

   (a) acute   (b) stuffy   (c) depressed   (d) sick   (e) exhausted

2. For three weeks I had been feeling very <u>dizzy</u>.

   (a) drowsy   (b) bloated   (c) ill   (d) terrific   (e) woozy

3. When I work late night, my eyes get <u>sore</u>.

   (a) faint   (b) painful   (c) groggy   (d) dim   (e) blurred

4. New breakthroughs would allow the cure of most <u>terminal</u> diseases.

   (a) incurable   (b) station   (c) extreme   (d) pale   (e) itchy

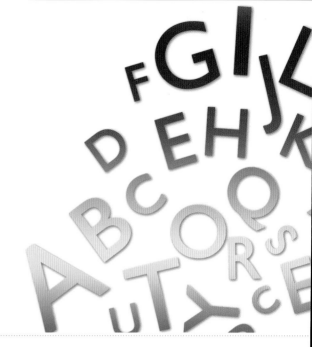

04

기타 건강관련
단어

01. ache

If you ache or a part of your body aches, you feel a steady, fairly strong pain.

My whole body aches. / I'm aching all over.

02. blind

Someone who is blind is unable to see because their eyes are damaged.

She started to go blind in her sixties.

I had my first blind date yesterday.

03. cramp

Cramp is a sudden strong pain caused by a muscle suddenly contracting.

I suddenly got a cramp in my leg while swimming.

04. deaf

Someone who is deaf is unable to hear anything or is unable to hear very well.

He's been totally deaf since birth.

05. exhausted

If something exhausts you, it makes you so tired, either physically or mentally, that you have no energy left.

I'm exhausted.

06. far-sighted

Far-sighted people cannot see things clearly that are close to them, and therefore need to wear glasses.

I'm so far sighted that I can't read the paper without my glasses.

07. limp

If a person or animal limps, they walk with difficulty or in an uneven way because one of their legs or feet is hurt.

Mario limped off the field with a leg injury.
He walks with a limp.

08. mute

Someone who is mute is unable to speak.

The president has remained mute about the project.

09. nap

If you have a nap, you have a short sleep, usually during the day.

Grandpa usually takes a nap after lunch.

10. numb	If a part of your body is numb, you cannot feel anything there.
	My fingers are numb with cold.
	My behind is still numb from my mother's spanking.
11. scratch	If you scratch yourself, you rub your fingernails against your skin because it is itching.
	Hannah scratched her mosquito bites.

EXERCISE 4

A 주어진 단어를 이용하여 문장을 완성하시오.

1. exhausted   (   )

2. cramp   (   )

3. numb   (   )

B 빈칸에 들어갈 알맞은 것을 〈보기〉에서 고르시오.

〈보기〉 scratched   blind   deaf   cramps   numb   limped

1. The most common cause of muscle _____ in exercise is lack of salt.

2. The victim's mother said she felt _____ over an arrest being made 30 years after her son was murdered.

3. The player _____ out of the filed with a knee injury.

4. The government turned a _____ ear to the warnings about imminent disasters.

밑줄 친 부분과 뜻이 가장 가까운 것을 고르시오.

1. China has been definitely <u>mute</u> over North Korea's human rights issues.

    (a) blind   (b) silent   (c) frostbitten   (d) fractured   (e) calm

2. He was completely <u>exhausted</u> after the marathon.

    (a) excluded   (b) worn out   (c) frustrated   (d) cast away   (e) displayed

3. She spread out a blanket and settled down for a <u>snooze</u>.

    (a) picnic   (b) festival   (c) doze   (d) tan   (e) joy

4. I had a terribly high temperature and <u>ached</u> all over.

    (a) threw up   (b) sneezed   (c) stumbled   (d) wept   (e) hurt

 Fill in the blanks with the correct word or expression form the list below.

> ⟨example⟩　fever – sore throat – scratch – chills – dizzy – diarrhea – swollen – allergic – faint – nauseated – vomit – sneeze – contagious – rash – bruise – runny – itchy – hangover

1. When I have a cold, I have a _____ nose and I _____ a lot.

2. Anne is _____ to some antibiotics. When she takes penicillin, her face becomes swollen.

3. Betty fell down when she was skating. She has a big, purple _____ on her leg.

4. I have a _____. It hurts when I swallow.

5. I can't get warm. I am shivering. I have the _____.

6. I have a stomachache and the runs. I have _____.

7. She hasn't eaten for two days. If she doesn't eat something soon, she is going to

   _____.

8. A mosquito bite is very _____.

9. Her temperature is 40 degrees C. She has a high _____.

10. When children have chicken pox, they want to _____ their skin because it is very itchy.

11. John twisted his ankle last week. It is still badly _____. It is twice as big as normal.

12. Cancer is not a _____ disease, but influenza is.

13. Yesterday he wore a woolen sweater. Now he has a _____ all over his chest. He is probably allergic to wool.

14. He had too much wine to drink. He feels very _____. The room is spinning. Tomorrow he will probably have a _____.

15. She has an upset stomach. She can't keep her food down. She is going to _____ again. She has felt _____ all day.

05

Compare dental terminology
and dental expression
for patient

환자의 눈높이에 맞춘 치과 용어 :
치과 전문용어와 환자를 위한 영어 표현법 비교

dental terminology	dental expression for patient	korean meaning
abscess	_____ in a tooth	
analgesic	_____ medicine / _____ killers	
anterior tooth	_____ tooth	
buccal	_____ side of the tooth	
calculus	calcium _____ on teeth	
carcinoma	cancer	
cariogenic	_____ producing	
carious lesion	_____ / tooth decay	
composite resin	tooth-colored _____	

dental terminology	dental expression for patient	korean meaning
crown	cap	
curette	_____ for cleaning teeth	
cusp	_____ of the tooth	
dental caries	_____ / _____	
dentifrice	toothpaste	
dentition	teeth	
endodontic therapy	_____ _____ treatment	
first molar	_____ – year molar	
fixed prosthesis	bridge	
gingivitis	_____ gum disease	
halitosis	_____ breath	
impression	_____ of the teeth	
incisor	_____ teeth	
injection	_____	
lingual	_____ side of the tooth	
malocclusion	misalignment of the _____	
mandible	_____ jaw	
maxilla	_____ jaw	

dental terminology	dental expression for patient	korean meaning
molar	_____ tooth	
occlusal surface	_____ surface	
oral	_____	
oral prophylaxis	teeth _____	
orthodontic treatment	_____	
pedodontist	_____ dentist	
periodontal disease	_____ disease	
periodontal surgery	_____ surgery	
periodontal tissue	gums	
periodontist	gum disease specialist	
pits and fissures	_____ in teeth	
pit and fissure sealant	sealant	
plaque	_____ on teeth	
posterior tooth	_____ tooth	
primary dentition	_____ teeth	
radiograph	X-ray	
removable prosthesis	removable denture	
restoration	_____	

dental terminology	dental expression for patient	korean meaning
root planing	_____ cleaning	
saliva	_____	
scaler	_____ for cleaning teeth	
scaling	removal of calculus and _____	
subgingival	_____ the gum line	
supernumerary tooth	_____ tooth	
temporomandibular joint	jaw joint	
third molar	_____ tooth	

A Odd one out – Three out of the four words in each line belong together. Underline the word that does not fit. Explain why the word does not belong.

> eye – nose – lips – finger – It's not part of the face.

1. ankle – toe – heel – thumb _____

2. shoulder – knee – wrist – elbow _____

3. heart – lungs – hip – kidneys _____

4. chin – calf – ears – neck _____

5. palm – tongue – thumb – fingernail _____

6. brow – lash – knuckle – eye _____

7. moustache – beard – eyebrow – nail _____

8. thigh – shoulder – calf – knee _____

9. liver – neck – kidney – stomach _____

10. lip – tongue – cheek – teeth _____

B Name the body part (There may be more than one correct answer)

> These are used for walking. legs or feet

1. This is used to smell. _____

2. These are used to chew. _____

3. This is used to think. _____

4. This is facial hair on a man's cheeks and chin. _____

5. These are used to pick things up. _____

6. This is used when you swallow food. _____

7. This is hair over the lip. _____

8. This connects the head to the body. _____

9. This joint allows your arm to bend. _____

10. This joint connects your hand to your arm. _____

11. This joint connects your foot to your leg. _____

12. This joint allows your leg to bend. _____

13. This is used to talk. _____

14. This hurts if you have a bad cough. _____

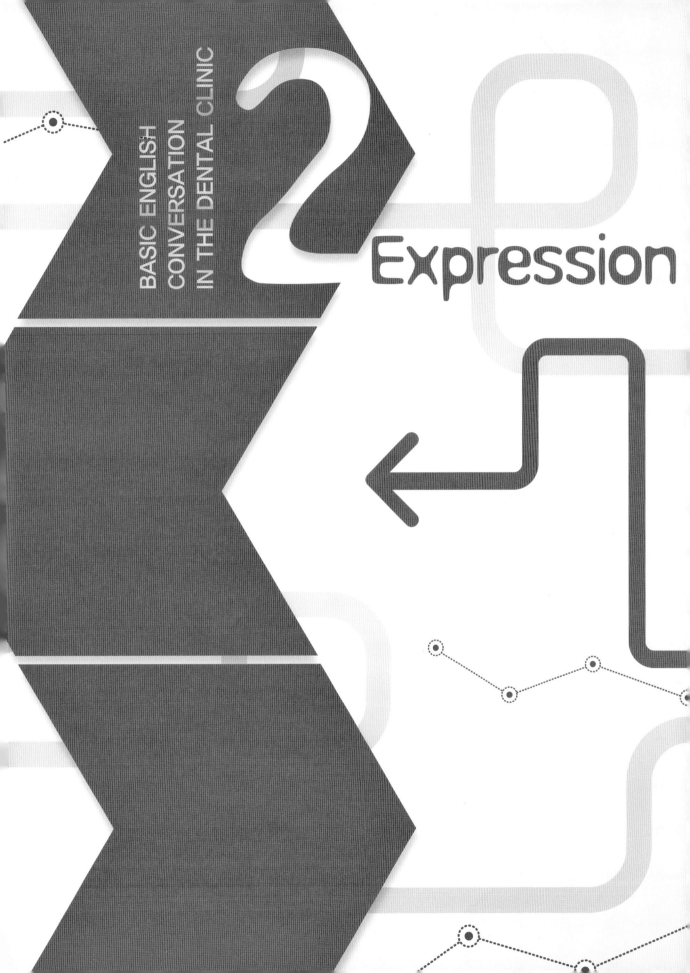

2

Expression

BASIC ENGLISH
CONVERSATION
IN THE DENTAL CLINIC

Intro

Part 2에서는 기본이 되는 영어 표현법을 숙지하고 암기한 뒤, 암기한 문장을 통하여 다양한 문장으로 표현해 볼 수 있게 했다. 간단한 표현방법을 구성해 놓았으므로 의료 전문가로서 기본적인 영어 표현법은 반드시 알고 있어야 한다. 따라서 기본적인 표현법으로도 외국인 환자와 원활한 의사소통을 할 수 있을 것이라고 본다.

01

Helpful
Expressions
for Reception

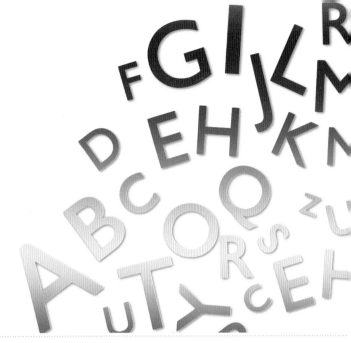

01. What can I help you?

02. Do you have an insurance card or identification card?

03. How long are you planning to live here?

04. What do you do in Korea?

05. May I ask who recommended our dentist to you?

06. Would you please wait for a moment?

07. I can help you immediately.

08. Please sit down on the dentist chair.

09. Lie down here. Let's have a look.

10. Have you ever been seriously ill before?

11. Put your head back.

12. Are you comfortable?

13. Relax and make yourself comfortable.

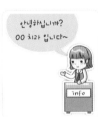

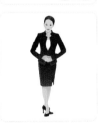

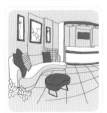

02

Dental History

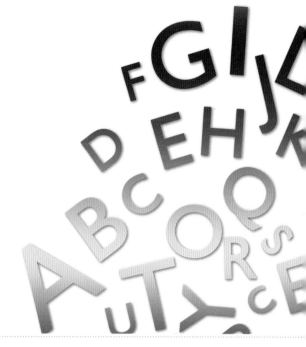

01. Reason for visit:

02. When was your last dental visit?

03. How often do you brush your teeth?

04. What texture brush do you use? (Soft / Medium / Hard)

05. Do your gums bleed while brushing?

06. Do your gums bleed when flossing?

07. Do you feel pain to any of your teeth when brushing or flooisng them?

08. Are your teeth sensitive to hot, cold, sweet or sour food / liquids?

09. Have you noticed any loosening of your teeth?

10. Does food tend to become caught between your teeth?

11. Do you have any sores or lumps in or near your mouth?

12. Have you ever experienced any of the following problems in your jaw?

- Clicking

- Pain (joint, ear, side of face)

- Difficulty in opening or closing

- Difficulty in chewing

13. Have you had any head, neck, or jaw injuries?

14. Do you have frequent headache?

15. Do you clench or grind your teeth while awake or asleep?

16. Do you bite your lips or cheeks frequently?

17. Have you ever had:

- Orthodontic treatment (braces)?

- Oral surgery?

- Gum treatment?

- Your teeth ground or the bite adjusted?

- Worn a bite plane or other appliance?

18. Are you satisfied with the appearance of your teeth?

19. Have you ever had an upsetting experience in the dental office?

20. Is there anything about having dental treatment that bothers you?

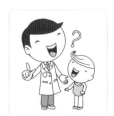 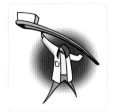 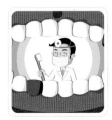 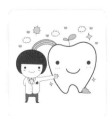

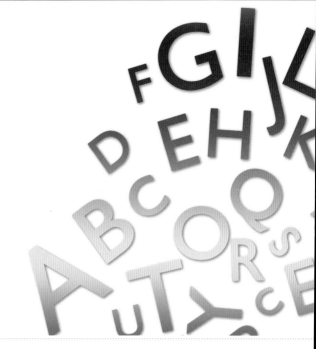

03

Helpful Expressions for Pain

01. What brings you here to my office this morning?

02. Do you feel pain?

03. Do you feel better than yesterday?

04. Where does it hurt?

05. Would you describe your symptoms please?

06. What kind of pain?

07. How often do you feel pain?

08. Is it a dull pain?

09. Is it a sharp pain?

10. Is it a throbbing pain?

11. Is it a constant pain?

12. Is it an occasional pain?

13. Do you feel a stabbing pain?

14. Does it hurt continuously?

15. Dose it hurt when you close your mouth?

16. Dose it hurt when you tap this tooth?

17. Is it sensitive to sweet foods, cold or warm temperatures or to direct touch?

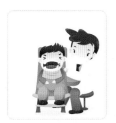 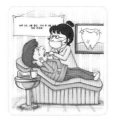 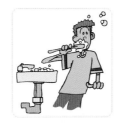 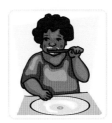

18. How about hot? (cold)

19. How about when you chew? (bite)

20. Now, I would like to check it.

21. Does it hurt where I touch?

22. How long have you had these symptoms?

23. How long has this been going on?

24. Let me take a look at it.

25. Please tell me if I hurt you.

26. It is nothing serious.

27. The diagnose is not confirmed and it may be nothing serious.

04

Helpful Expression
for Post Operation
care

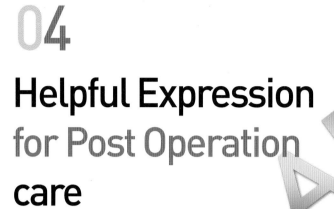

01. Put your head back.

02. Turn your head to the right.

03. Close your mouth slightly.

04. Open your mouth as wide as you can.

05. Are you comfortable?

06. Relax and make yourself comfortable.

07. Can you come back tomorrow?

08. Sorry for the wait.

09. Can you come on Monday in the afternoon?

10. Which is more convenient for you, morning or afternoon?

11. I'm glad to see that you're recovering very well.

12. Pleas call me if it swells or hurts.

13. Try to rinse out the spot where the tooth used to be.

14. Don't start brushing your teeth until tomorrow.

15. How long did it bleed?

16. It doesn't hurt now, dose it?

17. Take care of yourself. You'll be well soon.

18. Please let me know if the fever continues.

19. Try to eat lots of liquid food and avoid talking too much.

20. How is your appetite?

21. I'll give you an injection and some medicine to reduce the pain.

22. I would like to see you again in a few days.

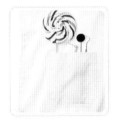 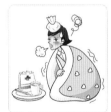 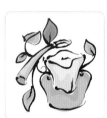 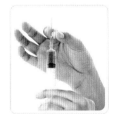

05

Helpful Expression
Radiology

01. X-ray examination is necessary for you to make a diagnosis.

02. The radiography will show me exactly what is going on inside your teeth.

03. Please follow me.

04. I will come to the X-ray room with you now.

05. I'll take an X-ray.

06. When was the last time you had a radiography?

07. Are you pregnant?

08. Is there any chance that you may be pregnant?

09. Grab the film with your finger.

10. Use your thumb to hold it.

11. Take off your glasses, Please.

12. Stand here and put your chin on the plate.

13. Hold the handles with your hands.

14. Don't move.

15. Please don't move until you hear a beep sound.

16. Thank you for your cooperation.

17. Come this way.

18. It will take about 5 minutes to develop the radiography.

19. Please wait for a couple of minutes for the X-ray film to develop.

20. The film will be developed soon.

21. I will explain to you after X-ray is developed.

22. The dentist will explain what is going on with your X-ray in more detail.

23. X-rays didn't show anything specific.

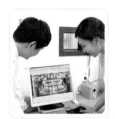
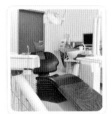
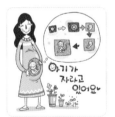
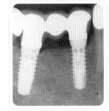

Reading
Comprehension

○ Intro

치과에서 흔하게 다루고 있는 치아우식, 치주질환 뿐만 아니라 구강예방에 관한 내용을 전문용어가 아닌 일반 환자들도 알 수 있게 요약정리하였다. 그리고 영어의 독해 향상을 길러 줄 뿐만 아니라 알기 쉽게 설명해 놓았기 때문에 간단한 문장을 익혀서 외국인환자들에게 쉽게 설명할 수 있는 능력을 키워보자.

01

Dental
Hygiene &
Dental Diseases

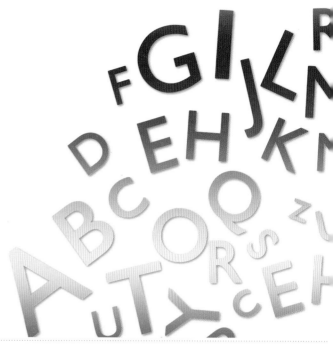

Most people have teeth which are one of the principal body's structure, also the teeth have very important function to masticate (chewing) food and prepare it for swallowing.

The tooth is any of the hard white objects in the mouth used for biting and chewing food. Dental hygiene meaning is connected with the teeth. People always should have something to eat and talk with a lot of colleagues in society.

Mouth is made up of the function which is the tongue, saliva, teeth and lips. Oral dental hygiene is very important because people have to eat and the mouth is always wet with saliva. Therefore oral hygiene is the practice of maintaining the mouth to carry out and prevent dental caries (cavities) and periodontal disease (gum problems).

If people do not care for their teeth, there may be a lot of plaque, bacterium and halitosis. Also this can lead to the loss of some teeth in extreme case. In addition some people who lost several teeth look like an old aged man and may be difficult to chew a particular type of food so that results in digest very hard.

For the various reasons, oral hygiene is necessary for all people to support the health of their teeth and mouth.

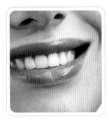 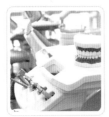

02

Compare Dental
Caries and Periodontal
Disease

The report illustrates that the biggest oral health problem is a dental caries and periodontal disease. Dental caries is the major cause of tooth loss in children, on the other hand Periodontal disease is the major cause of the tooth loss in adults.

A. Dental caries

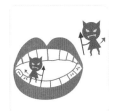 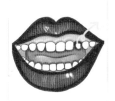 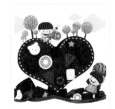 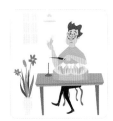

In dentistry, the disease is a hole in a tooth caused by decay, break down and damage (sugars, chocolates, sweet drinking and so on). Dental caries causes do not take care of teeth in preschool child group who have usually candy and sweet food. Thus, children should take care of their teeth for preventing the dental caries.

B. Periodontal disease

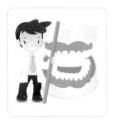 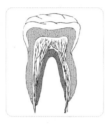 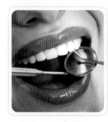 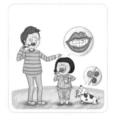

This is disease of the gums. Periodontal diseases occur usually in the over 35 age group who do not have health gum and alveolar bone. Periodontal care is more important it is because of supporting structure of the teeth. Periodontal disease is subjective symptom such as blood ooze throughout the periodontal area and the teeth are surrounded by plaque and calculus (tartar).

The progress of untreated periodontal disease: the gingival attachment recedes towards apical region of the tooth and then the tooth may have mobilized gradually after all it leads to lost the tooth.

03
Root canal
Treatment

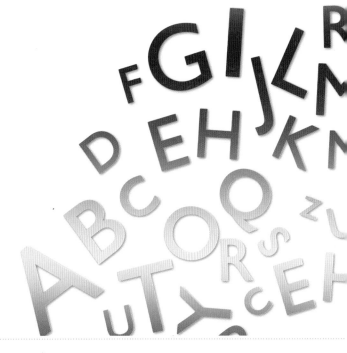

Root canal treatment, more precisely known as ENDODONTICS, is one of the recognized specialties of dentistry. The innermost layer of a tooth is known as the pulp. It is made up of blood vessels and nerves. Back teeth usually have more than one root, and each root will have one or more canals in it.

The pulp is normally protected by the outer layers of the tooth. When decay or a crack destroys the protective layers, the pulp is exposed to the bacteria in your mouth. This can result in inflammation, infection, and eventually, an abscess.

Endodontic treatment removes only the diseased pulp and returns the tooth to a healthy condition. It is also actually getting rid of all the infection from tooth. It is not going to be painful because the dentist is going to be giving patient the anesthetics. And then make sure tooth is numb before doing anything else.

Once the root canal treatment is completed, it is very important that the tooth be properly restored, not only for the function of your tooth but also for the success of the root canal treatment itself. For most back teeth, that means having a crown or other full-coverage restoration placed.

With modern techniques and analgesics, most people report that having a root canal is about as unremarkable as having a cavity filled. After treatment, over-the- counter analgesic should alleviate any comfort you may feel.

Endodontics enjoys a very high rate of success (90~95%), but no treatment on the man body can be absolutely guaranteed. For this reason, it is important that you return to this office for periodic checkups after the treatment is completed.

Patients understanding and cooperation are important parts of your endodontic treatment.

 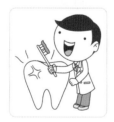 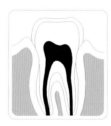 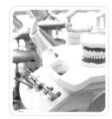

04

TBI & Diet for
Healthy Teeth

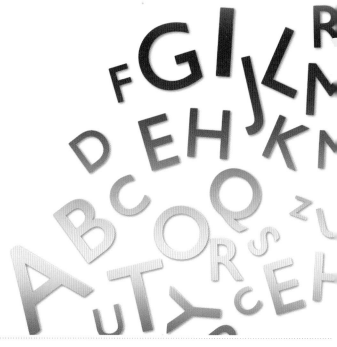

Dental hygienists suggest about TBI (Tooth Brushing Instruction) and diet for healthy teeth.

First, brushing teeth should be carried out regularly at least 3 times a day within 3 minutes after eating, for 3 minutes. Generally the toothbrush should have a short head, a flat bristle surface and a firm non-bending handle. Also, the toothbrush must be allowed to dry out completely after each use. A toothbrush should be replaced every two or three months and after illnesses, like a cold and flu.

Secondly, diet control is an important because people usually eat various foods. For this reason people should reduce all sugary food and soft drink to eat, because this food leads to dental caries. Healthy food for dental hygiene is fruits and vegetables. Also snacking celery, carrots or apples helps clear away loose food and debris.

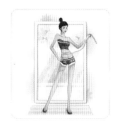
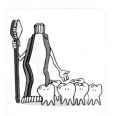
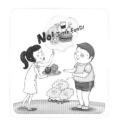
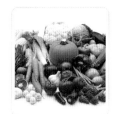

EXERCISE 6

A) What is the secret word?

Fill in the boxes with words from the word list.
Then, find the secret word and use it in a sentence.

Word List

plaque	cavity	apple	dentist
tooth	floss	brush	smiles

XXXXXXXX	B			S		XXXXXXXXXXX		
	L	A		U	.			
XXXXXXXXXXXXXXXXXXXX		A				L		
XXXXXXXXXXXXXX	F				S			
XXXXXXXXXXXXX	C				I	T		
XXXXXXXXXX		N	T		S	T		
XXXXXXXXXXXXXXXXX		O				H		
	M	L	S	XXXXXXXXXXXXXXX				

The secret word is

_____

sample sentence:

Yesterday I went to the dentist and had _____

placed on my back teeth to help prevent decay.

B Diet and dental health

What food should I eat?

To make sure that you are getting enough nutrients for good general and oral health, you should choose foods from these basic food groups each day:

> *bread, cereals, rice and pasta*
>
> *vegetables*
>
> *fruit*
>
> *milk, yogurt and cheese*
>
> *meat, poultry, fish, dry beans, eggs and nuts*
>
> *fats, oils and sweets – use sparingly*

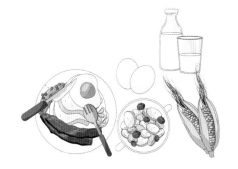

What food should I not eat?

When you snack, avoid soft, sweet, sticky foods such as cakes, candy and dried fruits which cling to your teeth and promote tooth decay.

Instead, choose dentally healthy foods such as nuts, raw vegetables, plain yogurt, cheese popcorn and sugarless gum or candy.

Preventive care

What brush?

Brushing your teeth after meals and between-meal snacks not only gets rid of food particles, it removes plaque, the sticky film that forms on teeth. Plaque is made up of bacteria that produce acids that cause tooth decay and gum disease, so thorough removal of plaque is the main goal of brushing.

Using a fluoride toothpaste is also important because the fluoride reduces bacteria levels, as well as remineralizes tooth surfaces, making them stronger.

Your dentist or dental hygienist can recommend the best toothbrush for you. Generally, a brush with soft, end-rounded or polished bristles is less likely to injure gum tissue or damage the tooth surface.

The size, shape and angle of the brush should allow you to reach every tooth. Children need smaller brushes than those designed for adults.

Remember: worn-out toothbrushes can not properly clean your teeth and may injure your gums.

Toothbrushes should be replaced every three or four months.

D Dental emergencies

Injuries to the mouth may include teeth that have been knocked out (evulsed), forced out of position (extruded), or broken (fractured). Sometimes lips, gums or cheeks have cuts. Oral injuries are often painful, and should be treated by a dentist as soon as possible.

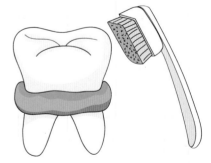

When a tooth is knocked out you should:

- *Attempt to find the tooth.*
- *Immediately call your dentist for an emergency appointment.*
- *Gently rinse, but do not scrub the tooth to remove dirt or debris.*
- *Place the clean tooth in your mouth between the cheek and gum.*
- *Do not attempt to replace the tooth into the socket. This could cause further damage.*
- *Get to the dentist as soon as possible. If it is within a half hour of the injury, it may be possible to re-implant the tooth.*
- *If it is not possible to store the tooth in the mouth of the injured person (e.g., a young child,) wrap the tooth in a clean cloth or gauze and immerse in milk.*

05

Wisdom Teeth that have
Emerged may Develop
Decay and Gum Disease

Often a person's Jaw is not big enough to accommodate the new molars when they begin to emerge. The tooth may fail to break all the way through the gum and instead become stuck in the Jaw. An impacted wisdom tooth has the potential to crowd other teeth or create painful, inflamed, and often infected, flaps in the gum.

Wisdom teeth that have emerged may develop decay and gum disease, because they can be difficult to clean. Most problems with wisdom teeth develop when people are between 15 and 25 years old.

Few people older than 30 develop problems that require removal of their wisdom teeth. Most dentists feel that people between the ages of 16 and 19 should have their wisdom teeth evaluated. Most dentists recommend that you do not wait until you are 20 or older to remove troublesome wisdom teeth, because the cones around the teeth continue to grow and harden. Extraction is more difficult and healing is slower for older adults.

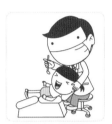
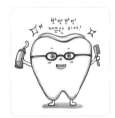
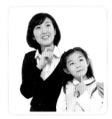
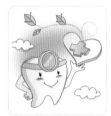

A # Fill-in the blank game

Use the following words in the sentences below.

⟨example⟩	brush	floss	molars	decay	plaque
	teeth	snacks	dentist	smiling	nutritious
	happy	visited	fluoride	sweet	sealant

1. It is important to limit the number of _____ snacks and eat more _____ foods.

2. The dentist said that _____ can help to strengthen the enamel on my _____.

3. Keeping my teeth healthy protects them from _____ and keeps me _____.

4. When I went to the _____, I learned how to _____ and _____.

5. When I _____ the dentist _____ were placed on my _____.

6. If I do not brush and floss to remove the sticky _____ from my teeth, and limit eating sweet _____, I can get decay.

7. A healthy smile is a _____ smile.

06

I Feel
Terrible

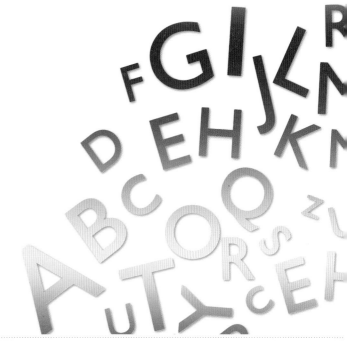

I feel _____ today. I have a _____ and a _____.

Uncle Wayne went to the _____ to buy some _____ for me.

I couldn't go snowboarding.

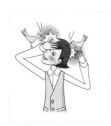

headache

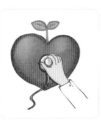

terrible

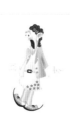

medicine

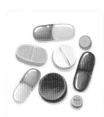

pharmacy

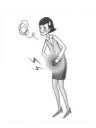

stomachache

1 Vocabulary preview

Look at the picture. Choose the best answer.

1. Marry feels ( ).

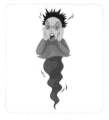   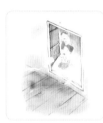   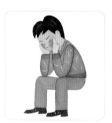

(a) terrible   (b) cold   (c) a headache

2. Uncle Wayne got ( ) for Mary.

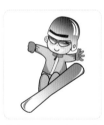   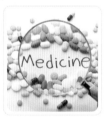   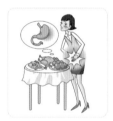

(a) a snowboard   (b) some medicine   (c) a stomachache

3. Uncle Wayne went to ( ).

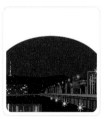   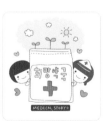   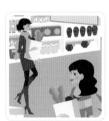

(a) River City   (b) the pharmacy   (c) the supermarket

2 Key expressions

Match the expressions.

☹ My head feels hot.　　　　　　　　(a) I don't feel very good.

☺ You'd better stay in today.　　　　　(b) Let me feel your forehead.

😐 You don't look too good.　　　　　　(c) OK, I guess you're right.

3 Dialogue

Read and fill in the blanks with the right expressions.

(a) You'd better stay in today, Peter.　　(d) I guess your are right.

(b) Well, you don't look too good.　　　　(e) I will buy some medicine.

(c) I don't feel very good.　　　　　　　(f) My head feels hot.

Peter :　Mom,　1.

Mom :　2.

　　　　Let me feel your forehead.

Peter :　3.

Mom :　Yes, your head is very hot.

　　　　4.

Peter :　5.

Do I need some medicine?

Mom :　Yes. Dad can go to the pharmacy.

 Questions answers

Circle the words you chose and practice with your partner.

1. (a) When was the last time you were (sick / tired / hungry)?

   (b) It's was (during the vacation / in April / last weekend).

2. (a) What was the matter?

   (b) I had a (hot head / stomachache / headache).

3. (a) What did you (do / eat / study)?

   (b) I (drank juice / took medicine / took a rest).

4. (a) Where did you (stay / go / sleep)?

   (b) I (stayed at home / played in my room / slept in Mom's bed).

5 On your own

A. Ask your partner. Write down their answers.

name	when?	what?	do?
Caroline	the weekend	stomachache	rest, drink water

B. Use the information above. Write about one of your partner.

My partner

My partner Caroline felt sick on the weekend. She had a terrible stomachache. She stayed at home and rested. She also drank lots of water. Now, she feels great!

6 Quiz

A. Write the letter with the picture.

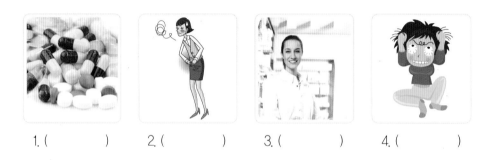

1. (   )　　2. (   )　　3. (   )　　4. (   )

B. Choose the best response.

1. My head feels hot.

   (a) You don't look too good.

   (b) Let me feel your forehead.

   (c) I don't feel very good.

2. You'd better stay in today.

   (a) I guess you are right.

   (b) I have a stomachache.

   (c) I feel terrible.

C. Fill in the blanks.

1. I don't _____ very _____ .

2. I _____ terrible.

3. My head _____ hot.

4. Let _____ feel _____ forehead.

5. I _____ you're _____ .

6. I'll get some _____ at _____ pharmacy.

7. _____ this medicine.

8. You'd _____ _____ in today.

9. _____ _____ a headache.

10. _____ I need some _____ ?

07

Visiting
the Doctor

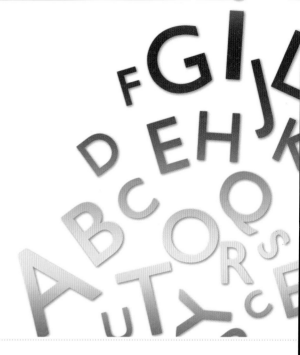

A. Look at the picture. Write the words under the correct picture.

| bandage | medicine | shot | sneeze |

(   )   (   )   (   )   (   )

B. Write the words in the blankets.

| fever | checks | coughs | stomachache |

1. The nurse (   ) on me three times a day.

2. Eric has a cold. He (　　　　　) a lot.

3. Lisa has to stay in bed today. She has a high (　　　).

4. I have a (　　　　　). I ate too much chocolate.

C. Write the words in the blankets.

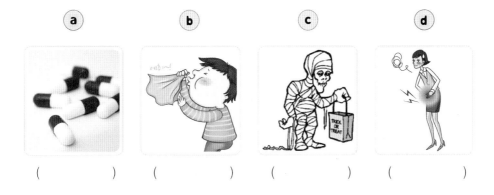

| a | b | c | d |

(　　　　　)　(　　　　　)　(　　　　　)　(　　　　　)

① Reading

A. Read the passage. Choose the best answer to each question.

Kate has to go to the doctor. Does she have a stomachache? No. Does she have a cold? No. Kate is getting a shot so she won't get sick. Kate thinks it will hurt. The doctor comes in. He tells her that it won't hurt. Kate looks away. Suddenly, it's all over. The doctor puts a bandage on her arm. Kate smiles. The doctor was right. That didn't hurt at all!

1. Why does Kate have to see the doctor?

   (a) She has a stomachache.

   (b) She has a fever.

   (c) She has a cold.

   (d) She has to get a shot.

2. What does Kate first think about the shot?

   (a) She thinks it will be fun.

   (b) She thinks it will hurt.

   (c) She thinks it won't hurt.

   (d) She thinks it will be fast.

B. Read the passage and choose the best picture for each question.

G : You don't look good, Chris.

B : I don't feel well. I'm sick.

G : Oh, no! What's wrong with you?

B : I am coughing and sneezing a lot. I also feel really hot.

G : I think you have a fever. You need to see a doctor. You can get checked out, and they can give you medicine.

B : OK, I will go see the doctor now. I hope I feel better tomorrow!

1. What's wrong with Chris?

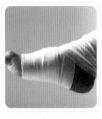

(a)

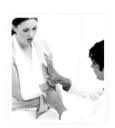
(b)

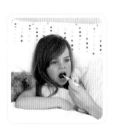
(c)

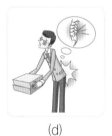
(d)

2. What does Chris need to get?

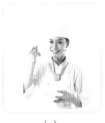
(a)

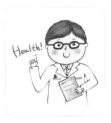
(b)

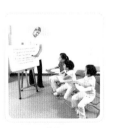
(c)

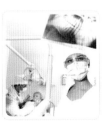
(d)

C. Read the passage. Then, look at the pictures.
Choose the picture that not belong.

Sho Yano is studying to become a doctor. He was only twelve years old when he started at the school for doctors. Now, he's eighteen. Soon, he'll be done with school. Then, he'll be a real doctor. Sho is a very smart boy. He also works very hard. Sho wants to help sick people. He wants to make new medicine, too.

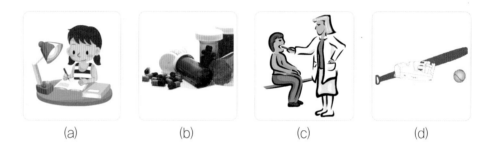

(a)   (b)   (c)   (d)

2 QUIZ

A. Match the correct response in each blanket.

G : What did the doctor tell you? (　　　)

B : It's three o'clock. Why are you still in bed? (　　　)

G : Why do you have to go to the doctor's office? (　　　)

(a) I don't feel well. I have a stomachache.

(b) I have to get my shots.

(c) He said I have a cold. He gave me some medicine.

B. Read and choose the best answer to each questions.

G : I don't feel well. I think I'm sick.

B : What's wrong?

G : My nose is running, and my head hurts. I keep sneezing, too.

B : That happened to me last week. I had a cold. Maybe you caught my cold.

G : I think I did. I need to go see the doctor.

B : That's a good idea. I hope you feel better!

1. Which is true?

(a) The boy is sick now.

(b) The boy needs to go see the doctor.

(c) The girl caught the boy's cold.

(d) The girl is coughing a lot.

G : Brian, what happened to your leg?

B : I hurt it. I was playing soccer. I ran into someone and fell.

G : That's too bad. I broke my arm last year. It hurt a lot. Does your leg hurt?

B : Not anymore. I went to the doctor. He said it wasn't broken. He put a bandage on my leg.

G : Well, I hope your leg gets better soon.

B : Thanks, me too. I want to play soccer again.

2. What happened to Brian?

(a) He hurt his leg.   (b) He broken his arm.

(c) He has a cold.   (d) He fell of his bike.

B : I went to the doctor today.

G : What's wrong with you? Are you sick?

B : No. I go to the doctor every year, even if I'm not sick.

G : What did doctor do to you?

B : She checked my eyes, my ears, and my mouth. Then, she gave me a shot.

G : Ouch! I don't like getting shots.

3. What did the doctor give to the boy?

(a) Some soup   (b) A bandage

(c) Some medicine   (d) A shot

C. Put the picture in the correct order.

One day, Mike was riding his bike with his friends. There was a big rock in the road. Mike's bike hit the rock, and he fell off. He was hurt. Mike began to cry. His mother took him to the doctor. Mike's arm was hurt. he had to wear a bandage. Mike couldn't ride a bike for a longtime. But he could still run around and play.

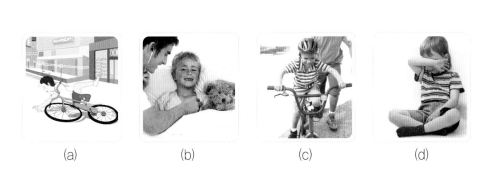

| (a) | (b) | (c) | (d) |

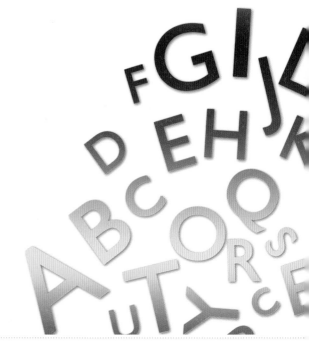

08

Health
and Safety

① Warming up

A. Unscramble the sentences.

1. ? / you / today / feeling / how / are

_____

2. take / she / going / your / is / to / temperature / .

_____

3. go / rest / . / and / should / you / to / bed

_____

4. has / . / sprained / my / ankle / sister / an

_____

B. Read and answer.

Recent research shows that children today are less healthy than children in the 1960s.

People think that being healthy means they are not sick. This is not necessarily true. Doctors and other health professionals now know that good health involves more. The healthiest people take care of their bodies and their minds. They eat well and they get regular exercise to strengthen their muscles, hearts, and lungs. They get enough sleep every night. They make time to relax and free their minds of worry.

Average Sleep Requirements	
Age	Hours of sleep in a 24-hour period
Newborn to 1 year	14~18
2~4 year	10~12
5~10 year	9~10
11~17 year	8~9
18 and up	7~8

1. Were children more healthy in the 1960s?

2. What should you take care of to be healthy?

3. How should you do this?

4. How many hours should you sleep?

2 Answer the fitness quiz

A. Discuss your answers in groups. (Yes / No, Suggestions)

1. Do you eat well?

2. Do you get regular exercise?

3. Do you sleep enough?

4. Do you make time to relax?

B. Read about Mandy the singer.

My name is Mandy. I am a singer. I like singing and dancing. I should keep fit. I should exercise for two hours every day. I like running and rollerblading, but I don't like swimming. I like fruits and vegetables, but I don't like water. I should drink eight cups of water every day. Last week I had a headache and a cold. The doctor said I should drink more water.

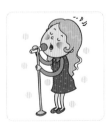

1. True or false?

(a) Mandy is a dancer.

▨ T   ▨ F

(b) Mandy should exercise for ten hours every day.

▨ T   ▨ F

(c) Mandy likes running.

▨ T   ▨ F

(d) Mandy shouldn't drink more water.

▨ T   ▨ F

2. How many sentences can you make?

Mandy should _____ .

3. What about you?

(a) I like _____ and _____ .

(b) I don't like _____ or _____ .

(c) I should _____ .

(d) I shouldn't _____ .

09

What do you know
about Healthcare?

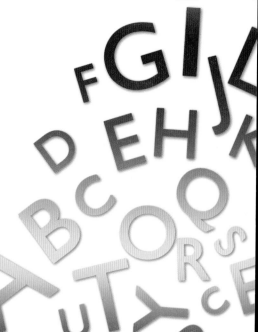

① Healthy life

A. Goal

Learn about illness and healthcare.

Learn health related vocabulary.

B. Example questions

✚ How does the man feel?

✚ How does the gril feel after the conversation?

✚ What is the attitude of the passage?

C. Warming - up

1. How do you think the person in the bed feels?

2. How do you think the man feels in the picture?

3. How do you feel seeing the picture?

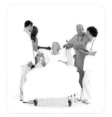

2 Guess what

What do you think the pictures are about? Number the pictures.

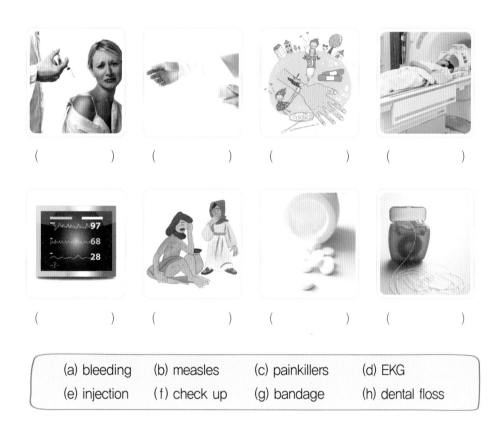

(   )   (   )   (   )   (   )

(   )   (   )   (   )   (   )

| (a) bleeding | (b) measles | (c) painkillers | (d) EKG |
| (e) injection | (f) check up | (g) bandage | (h) dental floss |

3 Let's talk

Let's talk more about healthcare.

1. What is the worst illness you've ever had?

2. What do you usually do when you are sick?

Reading

A. Read the passage and answer the questions.

We usually use painkillers to ease headaches, toothaches, and stomachaches, etc. Let's imagine this. One of your teeth in the back really hurts. You think you should go see a dentist, but you dread going to the dentist. You take a painkiller. You're much relieved, and can keep up your daily routine. Now every time you feel a toothache, you take painkillers instead of going to the dentist. It may be an easy way, but it can cause a serious problem. Your disease might get worse, or you may experience unpleasant side effects. Therefore, painkillers should always be used with the prescription only when necessary. And you should follow the instructions correctly.

1. What's the writer's attitude toward the use of painkillers?

(a) Painkillers are not helpful to reduce your pain.

(b) You need to use painkillers with the doctors's advice.

(c) Painkillers ar more beneficial than harmful.

(d) Painkillers decrease the chance of getting a serious disease.

2. According to the writer, why do people use painkillers?

_____

B. Read the passage and answer the questions.

Most cuts are usually minor, and most minor cuts stop bleeding on their own in about a few minutes. So they can be treated at home easily. First remove dirt in the cut and clean it with cool water. By doing this, you can get rid of the chance of getting an infection. You shouldn't use soap. Then dry the wounded area and you can apply antibiotic ointment and bandage the wound. You must keep the dressing clean by changing it often. However, if the wound is more severe and very deep, you should go to the hospital immediately. It may require stitching or further treatment.

1. What does the writer think about treating minor cuts?

(a) No treatment is necessary.

(b) You can easily treat them at home.

(c) You should see a doctor immediately.

(d) You need to stitch the wound.

2. Place the events in the correct time order.

(a) _____ Bandage the wound.

(b) _____ Remove dirt from your cut. ·

(c) _____ Wash the wound with cool water.

(d) _____ Apply antibiotic ointment to the wound.

C. Read the passage and answer the questions.

There has been an outbreak of the measles and many people are getting it. If you have the measles, the first symptom that you will notice is a skin rash on your neck. Other symptoms include a runny nose, stomachache and cough. You will feel tired and have difficulty eating and sleeping. These symptoms will last about seven days. There is no cure, but your doctor can give you some medicine that will help. The measles is usually not serious and will clear up on its own. But for some people it can be serious, so if you notice any of these symptoms you should see your doctor.

1. What is the tone of the writer's message?

(a) upset   (b) whimsical

(c) horrified   (d) informative

2. Check T(True) for true and F(False) for false.

(a) The measles is spreading quickly.

　　T   F

(b) There's no cure for the measles.

　　T   F

(c) In most cases the measles usually clears up its own.

　　T   F

3. Symptoms of the measles

_____   _____

_____   _____

_____   _____

D. Read the passage and answer the questions.

I know that it seems like a waste of time to come in for a check-up when you feel fine. But seeing your doctor for regular check-ups is an important way to find small health problems before they become big problem. For example, an EKG can find a heart problem before it becomes a big problem. Most of us are too busy with work or school to pay attention to our daily health. We often don't get enough sleep and eat a diet of fast food. Our modern lifestyle can lead to health problems. Seeing your doctor regularly can help you to remain healthy.

1. What is the writer's attitude towards check-ups?

(a) He thinks that it is a waste of time.

(b) He thinks that it is important for people to know.

(c) He thinks that most people already know it?

(d) He thinks that people will find it unnecessary.

2. According to the writer, which of th following is NOT true?

(a) Check-ups when you feel fine are worthless.

(b) A busy modern lifestyle can lead to health problems.

(c) There can be some health problmes what we aren't aware of.

(d) Most of us don't pay much attention to our daily health.

E. Read the passage and answer the question.

At State University, our nursing degree is a four-year program that is fully approved. In the first two years of the program, you will take foundation courses such as chemistry, biology, and physiology. After you have completed the first two years, you will begin your practical training as a nurse. During the last two years, you will spend most of your time actually working in a hospital with real patients. You will work under the supervision of doctors. During the final year of your training, you will be able to give patients injections and assist doctors as they treat patients. During my training, I was even able to do procedures such as apply casts to broken limbs. It was very exciting.

1. What is the writer's attitude toward the nursing program?

(a) skeptical   (b) enthusiastic

(c) miserable   (d) entertaining

2. What do students in the State University nursing program do during their first two years?

_____

3. Read and fill in the blanks. Then mark T(True) or F(False).

(a) The nursing program at State University is a four-year program.

▦ T   ▦ F

(b) During the first two years students assist doctors as they treat patients.

▦ T   ▦ F

(c) The writer applied a cast to a broken limb in her first year.

▦ T   ▦ F

4. Fill in the missing information.

Nursing degree : a _____ program

* In the first two years : _____

* In the last two years : _____

_____

* In the final year : _____

_____

F. Read the passage and answer the questions.

Even if you brush after every meal and use dental floss on your teeth regularly, you should still visit your dentist at least twice a year. When you see your dentist you are helping to prevent several dental problem. Of course seeing your dentist makes sense to help protect your teeth. Your dentist can detect problems like cavities when they are easy to fix. As people get older, gum disease is the most common cause of tooth loss. Your dentist can detect early signs of gum disease and treat it. Your dentist is also trained to detect serious problems like cancer. Oral cancer is the sixth most common type of cancer in the world. The key to surviving cancer is early detection, so see your dentist often.

1. What is the writer's attitude toward the subject?

   (a) indifferent   (b) recommending

   (c) annoyed   (d) entertaining

2. What are the three dental problems that the writer mentions?

   _____

3. Read and fill in the blanks. Then mark T(True) or F(False).

(a) You should see your dentist at least twice a year.

☐ T   ☐ F

(b) Oral cancer is very rare these days.

☐ T   ☐ F

(c) Once a gum disease starts, it is impossible to fix.

☐ T   ☐ F

4. Fill in the missing information.

Things to do to have healthy teeth a

Every day regularly

－ _____

－ _____

Dental check－up

－ _____

✚ can detect _____ → easy to fix

✚ can detect _____ → treat it early

✚ can detect _____ →

ex. _____ is the sixth most common one in the world.

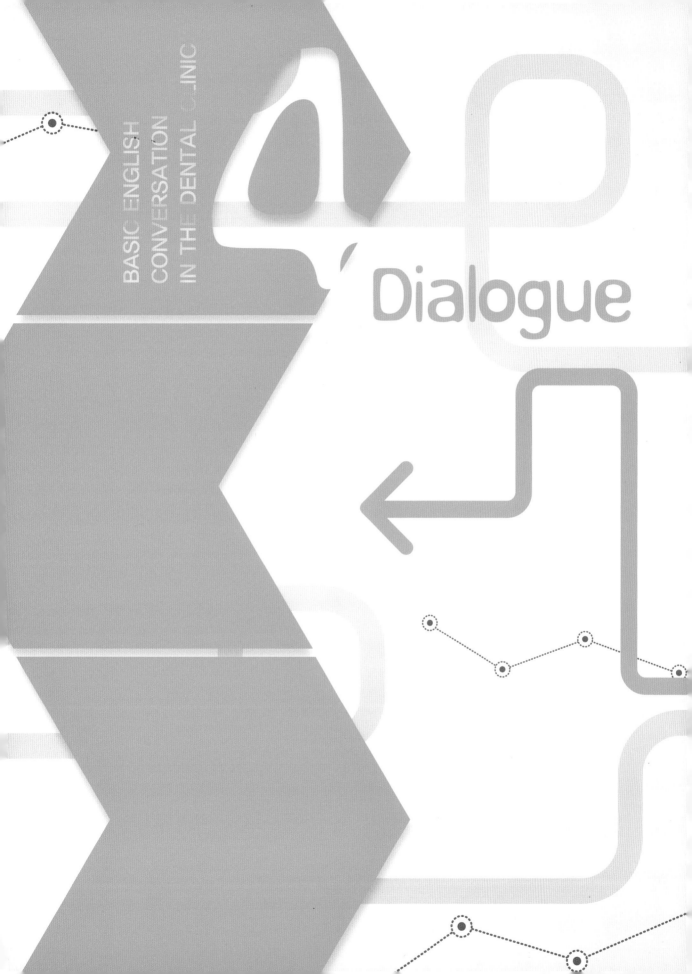

Dialogue

Intro

치과에서 일어날 수 있는 영어 대화방식이다. 대화를 통해서 외국인을 어떻게 응대할 것인지 알아야 하며, 대화체 문장을 통해서 조금 더 향상된 영어 문장을 구사할 필요가 있다. 예시로 나와 있는 dialogue를 바탕으로 영어식 대화체를 만들어 보자. 역할극을 통해서 영어 표현을 직접 소리 내어 보기도 하고 환자의 입장 또는 의료인의 입장에서 표현함으로써 영어 향상에 도움을 줄 수 있다.

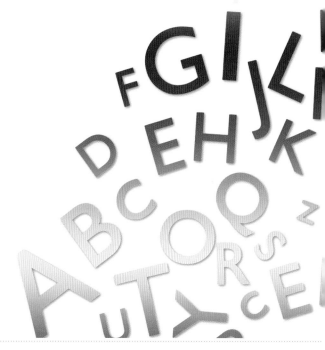

01

Dental English

1 Dialogue 1

Sam goes to the dentist

Sam **S**   Receptionist **R**

S Good morning. I have an appointment with Dr. Peterson at 10:30.

R Good morning, can I have your name, Please?

S Yes, it's Sam Waters.

R Yes, Mr. Waters. Is this the first time you've seen Dr. Peterson?

S No, I changed my insurance. Here's my new provider card.

R Thank you. Is there anything in particular you'd like the dentist to check today?

S Well, yes. I've been having some gum pain recently.

R Alright, I'll make a note of that.

S ......and I'd like to have my teeth cleaned as well.

R Of course, Mr. Waters, that'll be part of today's dental hygiene.

S Oh, yes, of course.

R Please have a seat and the Dr. Peterson will be with you momentarily.

S Thank you.

R You're quite welcome.

2 Dialogue 2

Dental check-up

Sam **S**   Dr. peterson **D**

S Hello, Doctor.

D Good morning, Sam. How are you doing today?

S I'm OK. Ive been having some gum pain recently.

D Well, we'll take a look. Please recline and open your mouth.... That's good.

S (after being examined) How does it look?

D Well, there is some inflammation of the gums. I think we should also do a new set of X-ray.

S Why do you say that? Is something wrong?

D No, no, it's just standard procedure every year. It looks like you may have a few cavities as well.

S That's not good news... hummm.

D There are just two and they look superficial.

S I hope so.

D We need to take X-rays to identify tooth decay, as well as check for decay between the teeth.

S I see.

D Here, put on this protective apron.

S OK

D (after taking the X-ray) Things look good. I don't see any evidence of further decay.

S That's good news!

D Yes, I'll just get these two filling drilled and taken care of and then we'll get your teeth cleaned.

3 Dialogue 3

Sam **S**   Gina the dental hygienist **G**

S Hello.

G Hello Mr. Waters. I'm Gina. I'll be cleaning your teeth today.

S Dr. Peterson has just filled two cavities. Why do I need a cleaning?

G Well, we have to make your teeth and gums clean and disease free.

S I guess that makes sense.

G Oral health leads to trouble-free teeth. I'll start off by removing plaque. Please lean back and open wide.

S OK, I hope it's not too bad.

G Everybody gets plaque, even if they floss regularly.
That's why it's important to come in twice a year for check-ups.

S Ah, that's better.

G OK, now I'll apply some fluoride. Which flavor would you like?

S I have a choice?

G Sure, we have mint, spearmint, orange or bubble-gum— that's for kids.

S I'd like to have the bubble-gum!

G OK. (applies fluoride) Now, let me give your teeth a final flossing.

S What type of floss tape do you recommend?

G Personally, I like the flat tape. It's easier to get between the teeth.

S OK, I'll remember that the next time I buy floss. How often should I floss?

G Everyone! Twice a day if possible!

Some people like to floss after every meal, but that's not absolutely necessary.

S (after finishing the cleaning) I feel much better. Thank you.

G My pleasure. Have a pleasant day, and remember to floss everyday at least once a day!

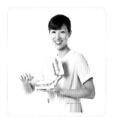
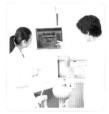
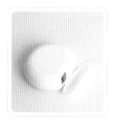
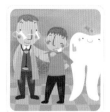

118

4 Dialogue 4

A. Have the tartar removed from your teeth every six months

Doctor D   Patient P

D What is your problem, Michael?
P There's a throbbing pain here in my mouth.

D Open your mouth and say 'Ah', Oh! the gum is swollen up.
P But I don't know why I have a headache, too.

D Don't mind it too much. It generally comes from the toothache.
P Umm.... two kinds of pains. It's like rubbing salt in the wound. My toothache is serious, doctor?

D It doesn't seem to be that serious.
P Then, I don't have to need an operation?

D I can tell you in more detail after an X-ray examination.
P How is the result, doctor?

D The swollen gum is not so serious, but you need to have a scaling.
P Scaling, Sir?

D Yes, the gum has swollen because tartar has not been removed.

Let me prescribe you some pills for the pain first, but don't fail to have the tartar removed from your teeth every six months.

P I see, Sir.

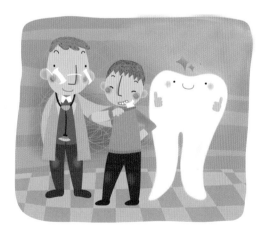

5 Dialogue 5

Scaling (Removal of dental deposits and calculus)

RDH. Lee   Julia

How are you? I am a dental hygienist. My name is Lee.

I am going to clean your teeth this morning.

Have you ever had your teeth cleaned before?

No, I have never had tartar removed since I was born.

Is there a lot of tartar on my teeth? Is something wrong?

Well, Open your mouth, and let me check first.

There are a lot of deposits behind your lower front teeth, and on the cheek side

of your upper back teeth.

I am sorry, but you don't brush your teeth well.

How come? I brush my teeth after every meal.

Tartar can't be removed with a toothbrush.

You should have your teeth cleaned once every 6 months.

I will explain how to brush your teeth well, and give you brushing instructions

after cleaning your teeth.

Please, make yourself comfortable. If you feel pain, please put your hand up. You might feel pain or it might start bleeding around your gums when I remove the tartar and plaque near your gums, but don't worry about it seriously.

Yes, I see. Please, make me comfortable.

(after scaling) I am going to polish the surface of your teeth. You are going to feel better.

I really appreciate it a lot.

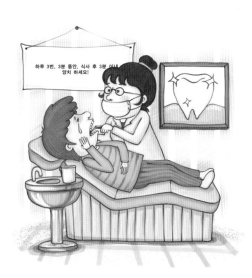

6 Dialogue 6

Fluoride in water

Nancy **N**   Alex **A**

N Hi, Alex, what did you do this weekend?

A Nothing too exciting. I had to write an essay for my chemistry class.

N Oh, yeah... what did you write on?

A Sodium Fluoride. It's one of the main ingredients of toothpaste. Many countries also put it in municipal tap water.

N Sounds pretty boring.

A You'd be surprised, but it's actually quite interesting and controversial.

N Really? Why's that?

A Well, it's highly toxic. If a small child were to eat the contents of a regular-sized tube of toothpaste, the child could die.

N Crazy! Why do companies use it, then?

A Aha! Therein lies the mystery of fluoride! It beats me. Officially, the companies claim that fluoride prevents tooth decay. However, researchers like Rebecca Carley strongly dispute this. She argues that the research on fluoride was manipulated and corrupted by the companies who funded the research. Apparently, research subjects had less tooth cavities because their teeth eventually fell out after prolonged use of fluoride!

N That's horrible! What about the use of fluoride in municipal drinking water? Is that dangerous, too?

A Well, sodium fluoride is a by-product of aluminum production. Aluminum manufacturers sell this byproduct to municipal water companies to avoid the high cost of legally disposing it. It's sold in big barrels with a label showing the skull and crossbones symbol and the warning, "Poison, not safe in any amount!" The chemical is then dumped into the water supply.

N How awful! I hope my tap water doesn't contain fluoride.

A Most English-speaking countries like the USA, Canada, Australia and New Zealand have fluoride in their water systems, but in Continental Europe and Japan it has already been banned. Can you guess what other products contain fluoride?

N No... not really.

A It's used in rat poison and in commercial insecticides, especially for killing cockroaches. It's also a key ingredient in anti-depressant drugs such as Prozac. Dr. Carley asserts that fluoride was first used in the prison camps of Nazi Germany and Communist Russia. It was used there to dumb-down the prisoners and to make them more obedient. Fluoride is also contained in certain processed foods and beverages.

N Well, thanks for the warning about fluoride. I'd better watch out from now on!

(Topic 1 fluoride in water)

A. What's the main idea of this conversation?

   (a) Fluoride is good for your teeth.

   (b) Fluoride is harmful and shouldn't be used.

   (c) Fluoride in toothpaste is okay but not in tap water.

   (d) Fluoride is only used in some countries.

B. What is NOT true about sodium fluoride?

   (a) It was used in Hittler's World War II prison camps.

   (b) Europeans have stopped using it in their tap water.

   (c) The use of fluoride is controversial.

   (d) Adults may safely eat toothpaste with fluoride.

C. How did big companies convince the public that sodium fluorid is safe?

   (a) By manipulating scientific research.

   (b) By selling it to municipal water companies.

   (c) By testing it on prisoners in World War II.

   (d) By putting warning labels on items for sale.

D. What may NOT be a result of educating the public about fluoride?

(a) Sales of toothpaste without fluoride will increase.

(b) More countries may ban the use of fluoride in tap water.

(c) Fluoride will be taken out of rat poison.

(d) People will avoid drinking tap water.

E. Read again to a part of the dialogue. Then answer the question.

> Q. What does the man mean by this:
> "Therein lies the mystery of fluoride! It beats me."

(a) He isn't really sure why the companies use fluoride.

(b) He thinks research supports the use of fluoride.

(7) Dialogue 7

Can you teach me how to floss properly?
-Instruction to the parents on taking care of their child's teeth-

Ms. Lee John's mom M

Children's teeth need brushing the time they erupt (at about six months of age). Although they should be encouraged to brush their own teeth, children cannot do a thorough joy themselves until they are at least six years old. Therefore, a parent must brush the child's teeth again after the child has finished brushing.

Between the ages of six and twelve the child may be capable of brushing his own teeth. However, the patent should check regularly to see that he is doing it properly. The same advice applies to flossing. However, most children cannot handle floss properly until the age of twelve. Therefore, this also must be the parents' responsibility.

John's mother is being instructed on how to care for her child's teeth.

L I have shown John and you how to brush his teeth. Now, it is your responsibility to make sure that he does it every day.

M John's mom: That is easier said than done. He always makes some troubles me when I tell him to brush his teeth before he goes to bed.

L He is properly tired at that time. You might have him brush his teeth earlier in the day.

M That's good idea.

L Also, you should brush his teeth again when he has finished since he will probably not be able to brush them properly until he is at least six years old.

M That sound like a lot of work.

L It is. But it's necessary. And don't forget to floss his teeth at least once per day. He probably will not be able to do his properly himself until he is about ten or twelve years old.

M Can you teach me how to floss properly?

L Sure. It's easy. First take about eighteen inches of floss. Warp it around the middle fingers like this. Here. (She hands the floss to Mom) You try it.

M Thank you.

L Now control the floss with the index fingers and thumbs, like this.

M This is easy.

L Put one index finger in the mouth, like this, and one outside.

M Ok.

L Now move the floss up and down about then times between the teeth to remove all of the plaque. You try it.

M Ok. ······. Gee, look how dirty the floss is.

L That's right. There was a lot of plaque between the teeth.

M Thank you for showing me how to care for John's teeth.

L You're welcome. That's my job.

8 Role play

- Make a group.
- Discuss any situation that could occur in the dental clinic.
- Work in pairs, take turns being a dental hygienist and a patient (ex: receptionist, dentist).
  - Who is A? Who is B?

9 Dialogue practice

1. Practice the dialogue in groups of two or three.
2. Take turns being your role and work with your partner.
3. Practice until you can do the dialogue without reading it.
4. Present it for the class.

02

Which Doctor Should
I Go to?

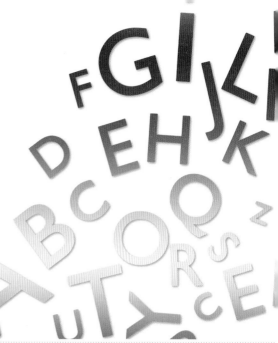

① Let's get started

A. Warm-up questions

1. What different types of doctors are there?

_____

2. When you ares sick, what kind of doctor do you go to?

_____

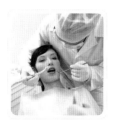 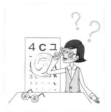 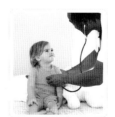 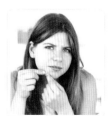

B. Vocabulary – Fill in the blank with the correct words.

| optometrist | cardiologist | zit | neurologist |
| disease | diagnose | treat (V) | pediatrician |

1. _____ to identify what a sickness is by medical examination.

2. _____ pimple: skin blemish.

3. _____ a children's doctor.

4. _____ to deal with and try to cure a sickness.

5. _____ a doctor for problems of the nervous system.

6. _____ eye doctors.

7. _____ sickness: illness.

8. _____ heart doctor.

2 Let's read

A. Reading practice 1

Tina 🅣   Joey 🅙

🅣 Hey, Joey. Where were you yesterday? I didn't see you at school.

🅙 Hey, Tina. I had to go to the optometrist.

🅣 Why?

🅙 I have been having trouble seeing things recently. In class, the white board is always blurry, and when I play baseball, I can't see the pitcher very well.

🅣 Oh, no. Well, what did the optometrist say?

🅙 He said I was nearsighted, so I need to start wearing glasses.

🅣 Nearsighted means you can't see things that are far away, right?

🅙 Exactly. I am going today after school to pick out some glasses. Want to come help me choose a good pair? It would be good to have another person's opinion, so I can find the best-looking ones. My mom said I can get whatever glasses I want, even the real expensive and fashionable ones.

🅣 Sure. Sounds like fun. Let's meet at the front entrance after school.
OK, but what time do you think you will be there exactly?

🅣 Hmm. It normally only takes me around ten minutes to get all my stuff together.

Let's meet at 3:40. Does that sound OK?

🅙 Sounds perfect. See you then!

Read and choose the best answer.

1. What did Joey go yesterday?

   (a) neurologist   (b) eye doctor

   (c) cardiologist   (d) pediatrician

2. What is joey's problem?

   (a) He is farsighted.

   (b) He can't see things that are far away.

   (c) His eye hurts.

   (d) He is blind in one eye.

3. Why does joey want Tina to go with him to the eyeglasses store?

   (a) He doesn't want to be lonely.

   (b) He likes Tina's glasses and wants her opinion.

   (c) Tin is an optometrist.

   (d) He needs help ti find a god pair of glasses.

B. Reading practice 2

1 A dermatologist is a skin doctor. Dermatologists help people who have skin problems and can treat different skin diseases. People visit dermatologists if they get burned or have problems with zits.

2 A dentist is a tooth doctor. Dentists help people keep their teeth clean and can treat tooth and gum disease. People visit dentists if they have cavities or a toothache.

3 A pediatrician is a special doctor for children. Pediatricians help young children and can treat lots of different illnesses. Children go to pediatricians if they have the flu or a stomachache.

4 An oncologist is a cancer doctor. Oncologists help diagnose and treat different types of cancer. People go to oncologists if they are worried they might have cancer.

1. Dermatologist

   (a) Definition _____

   (b) Job description _____

   _____

   (c) Reasonable to visit _____

   _____

2. Dentist

(a) Definition _____

(b) Job description _____

_____

(c) Reasonable to visit _____

_____

3. Pediatrician

(a) Definition _____

(b) Job description _____

_____

(c) Reasonable to visit _____

_____

4. Oncologist

(a) Definition _____

(b) Job description _____

_____

(c) Reasonable to visit _____

_____

C. Reading practice 3

Hi, students. Today, we are going to learn about a few different kinds of doctors. Many of you probably already know that there is more than one kind of doctor. But you might be surprised by just how many there are. In total, there are over 60 different types of doctors, and each type specializes in a few things. Let's look at a few of those types now. The most common type of doctor is a general practitioner. General practitioners are family doctors. They are the first doctor a patient sees, and they treat general sicknesses. Another type of doctor is a cardiologist. Cardiologists are heart doctors. They treat heart disease, and people who have had heart attacks. A third type of doctor is a neurologist. Neurologists treat problems of the nervous system. That includes any problem with the brain, spinal cord, nerves, or muscles. The final type of doctor I will talk about today is an obstetrician. They are pregnancy doctors. They treat women who are pregnant.

Read and take notes.

DESCRIPTION OF DOCTORS

1. General practitioners : _____

   They treat : _____

2. Cardiologist : _____

   They treat : _____

3. Neurologist : _____

   They treat : _____

4. Obstetricians : _____

   They treat : _____

D. Reading practice 4

Jeff 🌙   Mom Ⓜ

🌙 Mom! There are more! Every day there are more!

Ⓜ Jeff, relax. What are you talking about?

🌙 Zits, Mom. Every day I have more and more zits. You can hardly see my face anymore.

Ⓜ Oh, don't be ridiculous. Your face looks fine. It is normal for a kid your age to have a few zits.

🌙 No, it's not. None of my friends have this many zits.

Ⓜ OK. I don't think it's necessary, but if you want, I will take you to the doctor after school. Will that calm you down?

🌙 What can the doctor do about my zits?

Ⓜ Well, not the regular doctor, the dermatologist. Dermatologists are skin doctors and can give you medicine to help your zits go away faster.

J Really? That would be perfect.

M OK then, Jeff. I will make an appointment for us to go to the dermatologist today at 4:00 pm. Does that sound good?

J That would be great. Thanks, Mom!

M Now, can you finish getting ready so I can drive you to school?

J OK. Just give me five more minutes.

Read and check.

1. What is the main topic of the conversation?

☐ cause of zits   ☐ which doctor to go to

choose the correct statement.

1. (a) Mom thinks Jeff's face is fine.

   (b) Mom is worried about Jeff's face.

   (c) Mom thinks Jeff needs to go see the doctors for his face.

2. (a) The doctor will give Jeff cream.

   (b) The doctor will give Jeff a shot.

   (c) The doctor will give Jeff medicine.

3. (a) Jeff's appointment will be tomorrow at 4 p.m.

   (b) Jeff's appointment will be today at 4 a.m.

   (c) Jeff's appointment will be today at 4 p.m.

3 Let's talk

1. Which doctor is Joey? How about Jade?

What could be wrong with them?

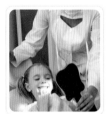 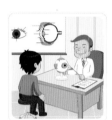

4 Read and number

A. Put the sections in order. (1~11)

(   ) A third type of doctor is a neurologist. Neurologists treat problems of the nervous system.

(1) Hi, students. Today, we are going to learn about a few different kinds of doctors.

(7) They treat heart disease, and people who have had heart attacks.

(   ) Let's look at a few of those types now. The most common type of doctor is a general practitioner. General practitioners are family doctors.

(10) The final type of doctor. I will talk about today is an obstetrician.

(   ) They are pregnancy doctors. They treat women who are pregnant.

(5) They are the first doctor a patient sees, and they treat general sicknesses.

( ) Another type of doctor is a cardiologist. Cardiologists are heart doctors.

(3) But you might be surprised by just how many there are. In total, there are over 60 different types of doctors, and each type specializes in a few things.

( ) That includes any problem with the brain, spinal cord, nerves, or muscles.

( ) Many of you probably already know that there is more than one kind of doctor.

5 Based Lessons

A. Match the words on the left with the correct meaning on the right.

1. G.P   (   )   (a) a person who checks your eyes

2. threat   (   )   (b) a doctor who performs operaitons

3. refer   (   )   (c) an emergency vehicle (car)

4. pediatrician   (   )   (d) a family doctor

5. obstetrician   (   )   (e) a heart specialist

6. psychiatrist   (   )   (f) a person who answers the phone and greets people in an office

7. symptoms   (   )   (g) give medical care

8. receptionist	( )	(h) a skin doctor
9. ambulance	( )	(i) a doctor who specializes in children
10. optometrist	( )	(j) tell about
11. cardiologist	( )	(k) a doctor who delivers babies
12. dermatologist	( )	(l) conditions of an illness
13. surgeon	( )	(m) send you to someone
14. describe	( )	(n) a doctor who specializes in mental illness

B. Match the sentences on the left with the correct follow-up sentence on the right.

1. He has a toothache.	( )	(a) He needs to see a psychiatrist.
2. He has a broken leg.	( )	(b) The surgery will be next month.
3. I have a bad headache.	( )	(c) The dermatologist gave me some cream.
4. She's pregnant.	( )	(d) He's going to the dentist.
5. He needs glasses.	( )	(e) You should put some ice on it.
6. I think he's having a heart attack.	( )	(f) He has a cast and crutches.
7. He is very depressed.	( )	(g) She goes to the obstetrician every month.
8. This rash is quite bad.	( )	(h) I need to take some aspirin.
9. He's going to have an operation.	( )	(i) The optometrist gave him a prescription.
10. Your lip is swollen.	( )	(j) I'm going to call an ambulance.

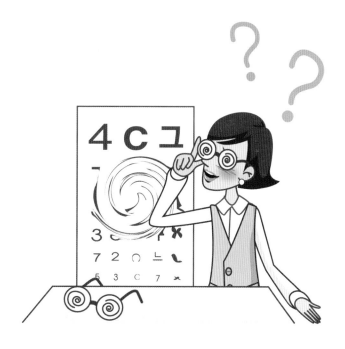

Intro

Part 5에서는 치아와 관련된 영어 스토리가 구성되어져 있다. 재미있는 에피소드를 통하여 간접적으로 영어 실력을 향상 시킬 수 있을 것이다. 딱딱한 소재가 아니라 흥미로운 주재가 영어 읽기를 유도할 수 있으며 간단한 영어문제를 통하여 단어를 익힐 수도 있고, 영어 이해력을 향상시킬수 있다.

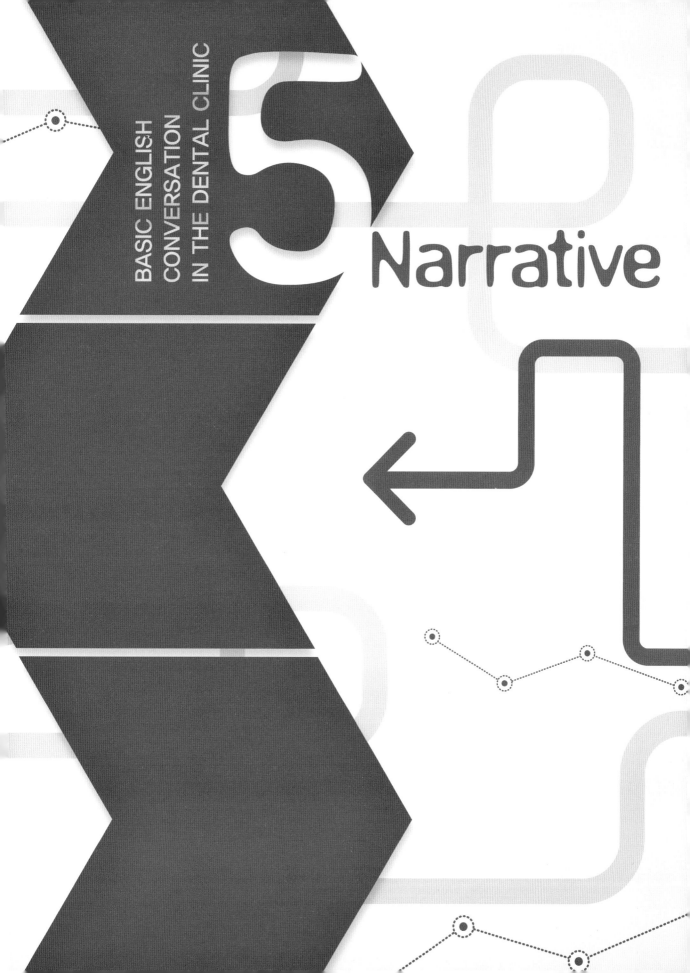

5

Narrative

01

I Hate going to the Dentist

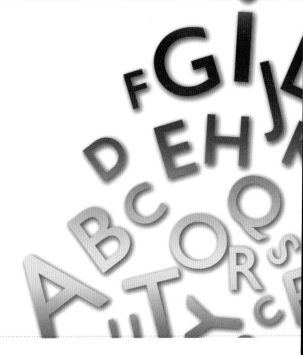

I run and hide when it is time to go to the dentist. I brush my teeth every day. But I still get cavities. Every three months I go to the dental clinic. It is a time for fear and pain. I hate the Dentist! It's not surprising that I hate dentist.

The office stinks. The lights are too bright. There are sharp-looking tools. There are little hoses that shoots air and water. They feel like a vacuum cleaner inside my mouth.

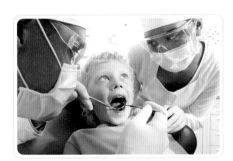

Last time, the dentist put his fingers and tools in there too. He started putting stuff in my gums. I couldn't say anything. I had this big needle in my mouth. I grabbed his hands. I almost jumped out of the chair. He said it shouldn't hurt. But it did. He kept shouting at me!

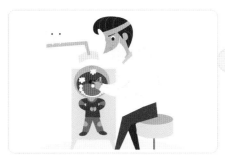 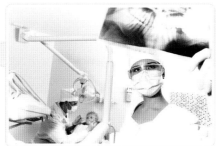

"Ron, sit still"

"Ron, your wiggling only makes it worse!"

"Ron, you need to brush more."

Then he reached for some gauze.

He had to stop the bleeding. It was the worst experience of my life!

Today my mother says the dentist has new things.

She says they are really cool. First the dentist rubs my gums. It tasted like candy. There's a wand. It looks like a ballpoint pen. It has a really thin needle.

"You can't even feel it," he says. "Pretty soon your mouth will numb."

"You will come home with a beautiful smile."

I hope he is right. For now, however, I still hate the dentist.

VOCABULARY BUILD UP

A Match the words to the correct definitions.

1. cavity   not able to feel

2. gums   to take hold of something or someone

3. grab   a special thin stick

4. wiggle   the flesh inside the mouth around the teeth

5. bleeding   something that happens to you

6. experience   the act or process of losing blood

7. taste   to be loose and move with quick

8. wand   to have some flavor

9. numb   a hole in a tooth

B Choose the best words to fill in the blankets.

1. You have a _____ . Do you have feel some pain?

   (a) stuff   (b) cavity   (c) tool   (d) mouth

2. His nose was _____ . I took him some tissues.

   (a) brushing   (b) bleeding   (c) numb   (d) building

3. When you brush your teeth too hard, your _____ hurt.

   (a) gums   (b) candies   (c) hands   (d) fingers

4. I _____ my tooth with my tongue. It was going to come out.

   (a) put stuff in (b) wiggled   (c) shouted   (d) hated

5. After swimming in the cold lake, my body felt _____ .

   (a) wiggled   (b) numb   (c) hot   (d) thin

COMPREHENSION CHECK UP

A Check true or false.

1. Ron does not have any cavities because he brushes his teeth.

　　▦ T　　　　　　▦ F

2. Ron likes the dentist at the end of the story.

　　▦ T　　　　　　▦ F

B Choose the best answers.

1. What does Ron think of the dentist?

(a) He hates the dentist.

(b) He wants to be a dentist like him.

(c) He thinks the dentist is the dentist.

(d) He wants to see the dentist.

2. What do the little hoses do?

(a) cut gums　　　(b) vacuum　　　(c) show teeth　　　(d) brush teeth

3. What is not true about the dentist's office?

(a) bad smell　　　　　　　　(b) too bright

(c) pretty nurse　　　　　　　(d) sharp-looking tools

4. What is not true about the dentist's new thing?

(a) taste like candy　　　　　(b) makes Ron numb

(c) wiggles Ron's teeth　　　　(d) has a thin needle

02
Meeting the Tooth Fairy

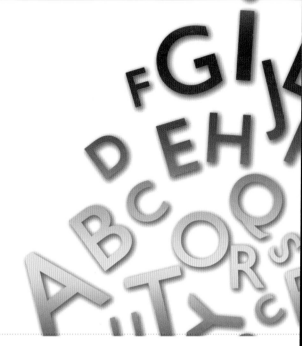

Claire ran home from school one day. She smiled at her mom. "Do I look different today?" "What do you mean?" asked her mom.

Claire smiled and asked "Do you see something missing?" "Missing? Your tooth!" said her mom and pointed at her mouth. Claire showed her mom the tooth. Mom said, "Well, I guess the tooth fairy will be coming!"

Claire went to bed early that night. She put the tooth under her pillow. She yawned and stretched. She soon fell asleep with her teddy bear Teddy. Claire dreamt of a pretty small fairy, She flew to Claire and show her a dance. Claire smiled at her and asked a question, "You gather missing teeth. Where do you keep them?"

The fairy stopped dancing and happily replied.

"I keep them in a pink cloud on the other side of the rainbow."

"How fantastic!" Claire shouted.

Suddenly something awoke claire in the night. It was a noise. She looked around in the dark. A light flashed across the room. Claire was scared. She hid under her blanket.

"What was that?" Claire wondered. Claire peeked out from the blanket. She saw the light again. It was flying across the room. It went under her bedroom door.

'Was that light the tooth fairy?' Claire asked herself. She lay in her bed. Claire felt something move under her pillow. She peeked under her pillow. Her tooth was gone. In its place was a shiny silver coin. She was so excited. She asked Teddy, "Did you see something?" Teddy said nothing. With her coin in her hand, Claire fell asleep.

In the morning, Claire looked at the coin. She wondered if it had all been a dream.

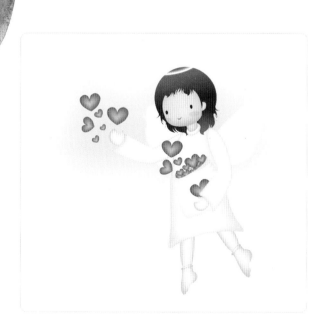

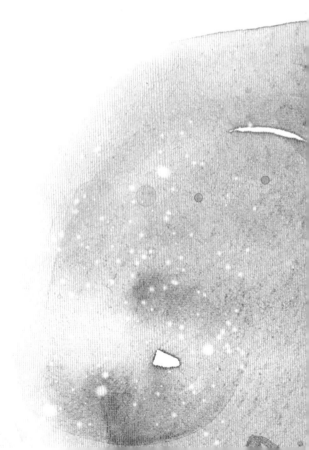

VOCABULARY BUILD UP

Match the words to the correct definitions.

1. missing	to go off to sleep
2. early	to look quick or secretly
3. yawn	to want to know something
4. fall asleep	frightened or worried
5. flash	to give off a bright light and disappear quickly
6. scared	lost; not be found
7. peek	before the usual time
8. wonder	to open the mouth wide while breathing in deeply

Choose the best words to fill in the blankets.

1. I have a _____ tooth. It is bleeding.

(a) different   (b) hard   (c) surprising   (d) missing

2. Something _____ . It was a shooting star.

(a) yawned   (b) wiggled   (c) walked   (d) flashed

3. Tim will _____ . His eyelids are heavy.

(a) peek out   (b) fall asleep   (c) play outside   (d) ask himself

4. Close your eyes. Don't _____ .

(a) go inside   (b) go to bed   (c) peek out   (d) make a noise

5. Fran was bored. She _____ and looked at her watch.

(a) missed   (b) asked   (c) wondered   (d) yawned

A Check true or false.

1. Claire dreamt of a tooth fairy.

☐ T   ☐ F

2. Claire found a coin under her bed.

☐ T   ☐ F

 B Choose the best answers.

1. What did claire and her mom talk about?

(a) classmates   (b) a missing tooth   (c) fairy tales   (d) last night

2. What did the tooth fairy not do?

(a) It was a song   (b) It made light   (c) It talked to Claire   (d) It went away

3. What did the tooth fairly leave?

(a) a light   (b) a tooth   (c) fa pillow   (d) a coin

4. Which of following was Claire's feeling at the end of the story?

(a) scared   (b) sleepy   (c) unhappy   (d) curious

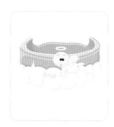
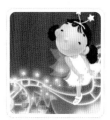

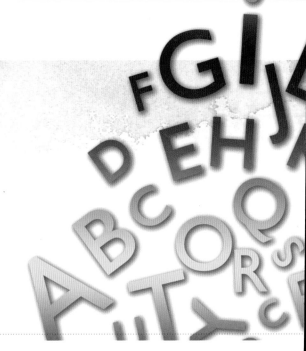

03

Arthur's Tooth

_Marc Brown

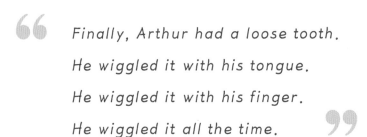

> *Finally, Arthur had a loose tooth.*
> *He wiggled it with his tongue.*
> *He wiggled it with his finger.*
> *He wiggled it all the time.*

One afternoon while Arthur was wiggling his tooth during math, he heard a loud scream.

Francine jumped up.

"My tooth just fell out on my desk!" she cried.

"Class, how many of you have lost a tooth?" asked Mr. Marco.

Everyone but Arthur raised their hands.

When Arthur got home, he didn't want any milk and cookies.

"What's the matter, Arthur?" his mother asked.

"I'm the only one in my class who still has all his baby teeth," he complained.

"Don't worry," said his sister, D.W. "Before you know it, all your teeth will fall out and you can get false teeth like Grandma Thora."

Arthur persuaded Father to make a special dinner for him: steak, corn on the cob, and peanut brittle.

"I can't believe one little tooth can take so long to fall out," said Father.

The next day, Muffy brought in a whole jar of her teeth for show-and-tell.

"I got two dollars for each one," she said.

"One from my dad and one from my mom. I put it all in the bank to earn interest. I'm waiting for my investment to double."

"Not me," said Francine. "I'm spending mine."

Later the class saw a movie called Nasty Mr. Tooth Decay.

"Between the ages of four and seven," the announcer began, "everyone begins to lose their deciduous, or baby, teeth."

"Everyone except Arthur!" shouted Francine.

The whole class laughed.

Arthur slid down in his seat. He wiggled his tooth as hard as he could.

In the cafeteria, Francine practiced her new tricks.

"Look!" she said. "I can keep my teeth closed, and still drink through a straw. And I can squirt water, too. Everybody line up for a squirting contest? Everybody except Arthur. Babies with baby teeth can't squirt water."

By the next day, Arthur was convinced his loose tooth would never fall out.

His friends tried to help.

Buster brought carrots for Arthur's lunch.

Sue Ellen showed Arthur how to put raisins over his teeth to make it look as if some were missing.

The Brain invented a special machine.

"It's a tooth remover," he explained.

"Just put your head in here."

Even Binky Barnes wanted to help.

"I can knock that tooth out in one second flat," he said.

That night Arthur spent a lot of time in front of the bathroom mirror.

He got up very early the next morning to wiggle his tooth again.

"See how much looser it is!"

He told his parents.

"That's it," said his mother.

"You need professional help. You're going to the dentist. Today."

"Going to the dentist?" asked Francine.

"Boy, do I feel sorry for you!"

There were other patients waiting to see Dr. Sozio.

"Sorry," said the nurse. "We're running late. Have a seat."

"Arthur, you were smart to bring a book," said Mother.

Finally it was Arthur's turn.

"I wish all my patients were as good at waiting as you are," said Dr. Sozio. "How old are you now, Arthur?"

"Seven," said Arthur. "And I still have all my baby teeth."

"I was eight before I lost my first tooth," said Dr. Sozio. "Everyone is different."

"Really?" said Arthur.

Dr. Sozio examined Arthur's loose tooth.

"This one should fall out very soon," he said.

"Just wait."

Arthur got back to school just in time for recess.

"Still have all your baby teeth?" Francine asked.

"Then you can't be in the game. I'm the tooth fairy. Only people who have lost teeth can play."

"If you're the tooth fairy," said Arthur,

"I think I'll keep all my teeth. I can wait."

He started over to the softball game.

"Whoever I touch," said Francine, "loses a tooth."

She flapped her arms.

"The one who loses the most, wins."

Francine twirled around and touched Buster.

She twirled faster, and touched Sue Ellen.

Twirling even faster, she slipped and hit Arthur.

"Sorry, Arthur," Francine said. "But I told you, no babies allowed."

Arthur picked up his glasses.

"It's OK," he said. "It's probably the nicest thing you've ever done for me."

"What do you mean?" asked Francine.

Arthur just smiled.

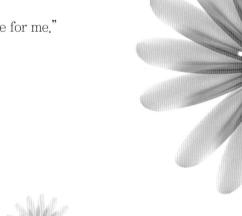

9

Writing

자기 소개서와 이력서를 영어로 써보자. 영작이라 부담감이 될 수도 있겠지만 겁먹을 필요는 없다. 영어로 적어 봄으로써 스스로의 영어 실력을 체크해 볼 수도 있다. 이력서는 본 책에 구성된 길잡이에 따라 한 단계씩 적어 보면 결코 어려운 작업이 아닐 것이다. 자기소개서 또한 서론, 본론, 결론으로 나누어 큰 덩어리에서 작은 덩어리로 구체적으로 적어 봄으로써 영어 영작의 완성단계에 이를 수 있다.

01

Cover letter
(RESUME)

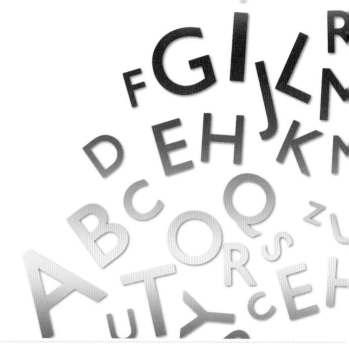

Clinical Hygiene Experience

January 2012 – July 2010 (part time or full time) – AAA Dental clinic

Education

Acquisition dental hygienist license
February 2012 – BBB University, Bachelor of Science in Dental Hygiene
February 2008 – CCC High School graduation

Computer experience

Digital Radiography, Digital Intra – Oral Radiography
Microsoft Word, Excel and power point

Periodontal / Clinical skills

Scaling and Root Planing
Making Temporary Crown (cap)

Leadership experience

Head of the hygiene department

02

A letter of
Self-Introduction

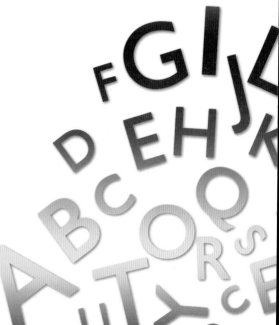

Short eassy organization

An effective essay must have the following elements.

Introduction

A hook is an opening sentence that attracts the reader's attention.
The sentence after hook gives background information necessary to understand the topic.
The last sentence in the introduction, the thesis statement, is very important because it gives the topic and the controlling idea of the entire essay.

Body paragraph

An essay has at least one body paragraph in which the writer develops the thesis statement from the introduction. The body paragraph begins with a topic sentence, followed by supporting details.

Conclusion

An essay ends with a conclusion that summarizes or restates the main idea in the thesis statement.

Sample 1

I would like to tell you about myself.

My name is Gil Dong Hong. I am applying for this dental hospital because. I hear this hospital has an excellent reputation, which is very warm like a family atmosphere.

I am a dental hygienist. I graduated from SS University at the top of my class. My major is dental hygiene. I have always worked hard to have good grades. I am interested in studying dental hygiene. I am also involved in many different activities such as tennis. I was the captain of the tennis club.

There are four members in my family, my father, mother, younger sister and myself. My family is very precious to me.

My hobbies are listening to K-pop music and making cookies. I love to share delicious cookies that I make with my classmates. When I am free, I usually go shopping and enjoy gardening.

Someone asked me what is my personality like? I can answer confidently. I am energetic and warm. I like to take care of patients because I am also thoughtful.

If I get the opportunity to work here, I will do my best. I really want to work together. If you choose me, you will never regret working together with me.

Sample 2

Let me introduce myself.

I am Min Ah Kim.

I study dental hygiene at Korea University. I want to get my dental hygienist license. So I study very hard now.

I would like to work at the New York Dental group in KimHae.

If I have an opportunity to work for this New York Dental group, I will do my best as a dental hygienist.

One day, I would like to work at dental clinics in New York, I know that I have to speak fluent English.

I wish to improve my English skills. I think that English really is a global language. I still study English after graduation.

I would like to be a professional dental hygienist.

I really want to work at New York Dental group with dentists and my seniors.

Thank you very much.

Write anything about yourself in English.

Example : Hobbies, what you like, or do not like, your hopes, favorite things and so on, everything of yourself.

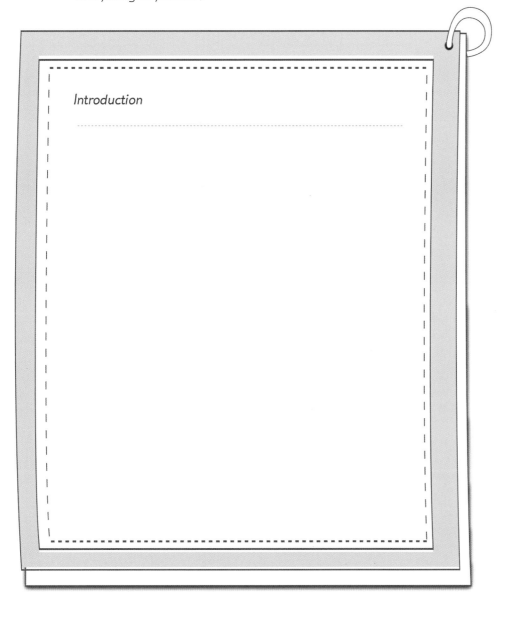

Introduction

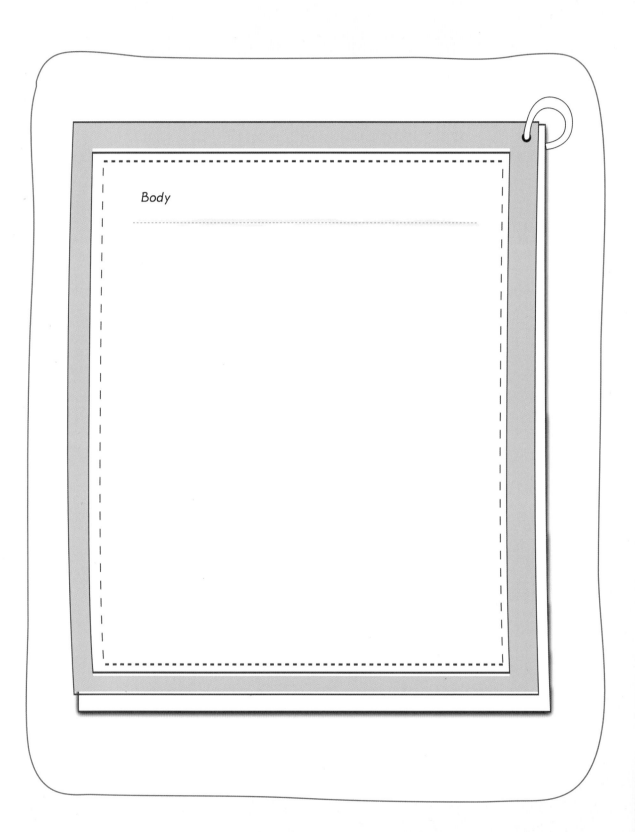

Body

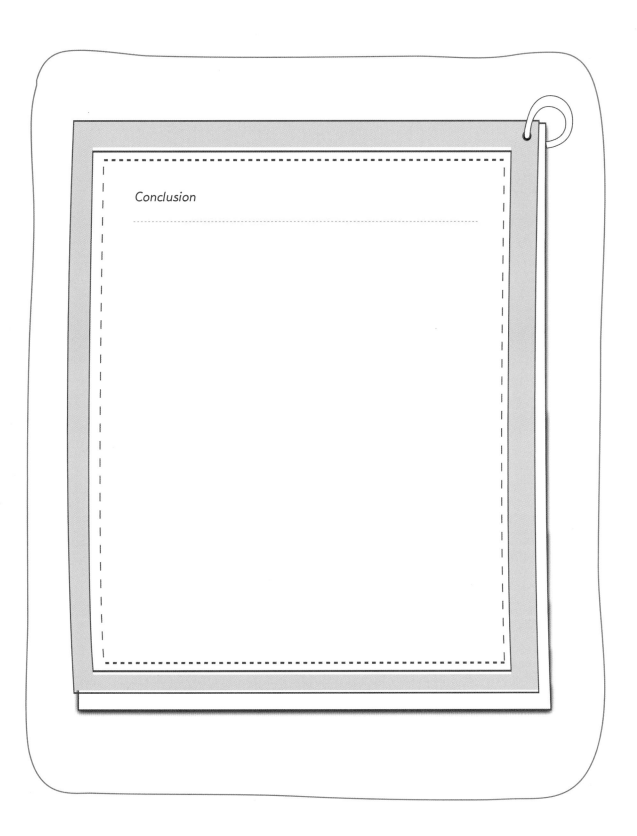

Conclusion

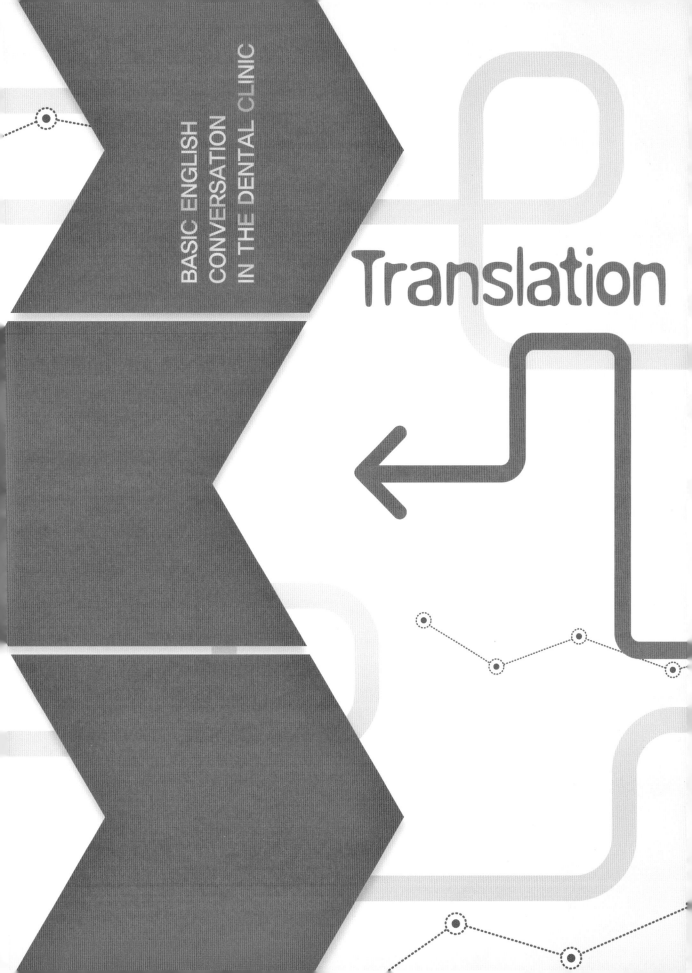

BASIC ENGLISH CONVERSATION IN THE DENTAL CLINIC

Translation

1. Vocabulary

01. 병원에서 사용하는 단어 I

1. 침: 침은 치과 치료 후에 고통을 완화시키는 것을 보여주었다.

2. 항체: 모유로부터 항체는 아기의 장과 연결되어 있고 감염을 막아준다.

3. 인공적인: 인공심장은 그들이 심장이식을 받을 때까지 환자가 살아있게 유지 시켜준다.

4. 항생제: 항생제는 세균이 초래하는 질병에 대항하는 가장 효과적인 무기이다.

5. 부검: 의학적 부검은 범죄현장에서 사용되는 또 다른 도구이다.

6. 정신을 잃다: 운전자는 아마도 운전 중에 정신을 잃었다.

7. 헌혈: 기증자가 건강하기만 하다면 헌혈에 나이 제한은 없다.

8. 멍: 다행히도 나는 서너 군데의 멍과 부운 입술이 전부였다.

9. 혹, 부딪히다: 그녀는 종업원과 부딪히면서 손님들에게 쟁반에 있던 음식을 쏟고 말았다.

   팀은 머리에 혹이 생겼다.

10. 화상: 아이는 화재로 심한 화상을 입었다.

11. 아파서 전화하다: 그는 오늘 아프다. 그는 오늘 아파서 전화했다.

12. 돌보다: 아이들은 친척에 의해 돌보아 졌다.

13. 시행하다: 병원에서는 그녀의 신장에 무슨 문제가 있는지를 알아내려고 임상실험을 시행하고 있다.

14. 충치: 그녀는 최근에 아래 어금니 중 충치가 하나 발견되었다.

15. 정기검진: 그녀는 정기검진을 위해 치과로 간다.

16. 목에 걸리다, 목이 메다, 질식하다: 어린이들에게 있어 땅콩이 목에 걸릴 수 있다.

   여섯 명의 사람들은 연기에 질식했다. 굶주린 아이들의 그림은 나를 목이 메이게 한다.

17. 병에 걸리다: 빈민가에 사는 여성들은 시골에 사는 여성들보다 HIV/AIDS에 걸릴 가능성이 더 높다.

18. 시행하다: 우리는 우리가 사용하는 물품에서 해로운 가스가 방출하는지를 알아보기 위해 방출 테스트를 시행한다.

19. 인지하는: 오늘날 많은 사람들이 본인이 낭비하는 것에 대해 무슨 일이 일어나고 있는지 잘 인지하고 있다.

20. 감염성 있는: 내 병은 전염성이 있나요? 나는 격리 될 필요가 있나요?

21. 전염되다: 그는 곤충 물린 자국을 통해서 말라리아에 감염된 것 같다.

22. 사망: 그 집은 너의 어머니가 돌아가신 후 너의 것이 될 것이다.

23. 교정 장치: 내가 십대였을 때, 나는 삐뚤삐뚤한 치아를 위해 교정장치를 착용해야만 했다.

24. 진단하다: 이모와 나의 가장 친한 친구의 엄마가 최근에 유방암 진단을 받았다.

25. 장애가 있는: 그 사고는 그에게 심각한 장애를 남겼다.

26. 질병: 질병의 증상 중 하나는 고열도 있다.

27. 1회 복용량: 그 설명서에 하루에 세 번 약을 먹어야 한다고 적혀 있다.

28. 안락사: 대부분의 나라에서 안락사는 여전히 불법이다.

29. 응급사태: 그의 가족에게 응급사태가 생겨서 오늘 결석할 거에요.

30. 검진하다: 한 의사는 나의 등을 검진하더니 수술을 받아야 한다고 제안했다.

31. 실험: 동물에 관한 실험은 금지되어야만 한다.

32. 기절하다: 그녀는 이글거리는 태양빛에 정신을 잃었다.

　　　나는 배고픔에 쓰러질 것 같다.

33. 치명적인: 그녀는 머리에 치명적인 상처를 입었다.

　　　대표의 주장에는 몇 개의 치명적인 결함이 있다.

34. 충전: 금 충전은 씹는 힘에 견디기에는 충분한 내구성이 있다.

35. 응급처치: 너는 학교에서 응급처치를 배운 적이 있니?

36. 건강: 나는 건강을 유지하기 위해서 조깅을 한다.

37. 골절: 그는 오토바이 사고로 복잡한 골절을 입었다.

38. 동상: 나는 동상과 다른 상처들로 인해 극심한 고통을 느꼈다.

02. 병원에서 사용하는 단어 II

1. 세균: 폐렴은 많은 수의 세균에 의해 초래될 수 있는 폐 감염이다.

　　쥐나 파리는 세균을 옮기기 때문에 박멸되어야 한다.

2. 좋아지다: 네가 빨리 좋아져서 정말 기쁘다.

3. 장애가 있는: 그의 본보기는 장애가 있는 사람이나 건강한 사람 모두 불가능을 가능하도록 용기를 주고 있다.

4. 숙취: 그는 아침에 숙취가 있는 것 같다.

5. 건강보험: 모든 국민은 국민건강보험이 적용된다.

6. 입원하다: 나의 아내는 교통사고로 입원하였다.

7. 예방접종: 당신이 저에게 간염예방접종을 해줄 수 있나요?

8. 중환자실: 모든 환자들이 집중치료를 받는 것은 불가능하다.

9. 감염: 감염의 위험을 줄이기 위해서 상처에 붕대를 감아라.

　아이들 모두는 정체불명의 바이러스에 감염되어 졌다.

10. 염증: 이 주사는 통증과 염증을 줄여 줄 것이다.

11. 주사: 이 약은 주사로 투여되기도 합니다.

　의사는 나에게 진통제 주사를 주었다.

12. 상처 입은: 그는 다리를 쉬게 하기 위해 누워 있도록 지시받았다.

13. 상처: 몇몇 승객들은 기차 충돌에 심각한 상처를 입었다.

14. 정맥주사: 정맥주사가 그녀의 침대 옆에 걸려있다.

15. 약: 당신은 어떤 약을 먹나요?

　그는 신장을 위한 약물치료를 받고 있다.

16. 정신적인: 시간이 지남에 따라, 그녀의 육체적 그리고 정신적 건강이 나빠졌다.

17. 비만: 비만은 지방의 양이 과도하게 많은 것으로 정의되어 있다.

18. 연고: 당신은 연고를 발라야 한다.

19. 수술: 그는 그의 어깨 수술을 했다.

　그들은 그에게 수술을 할 예정입니까?

20. 장기: 만약 장기 기증자로써 스스로 등록한다면 당신은 많은 사람의 삶을 살릴 수 있을 것이다.

21. 처방전 없는 약: 처방전 없이 살 수 있는 약을 남용하는 10대와 청소년이 있다.

22. 마비하다: 그는 말에서 떨어졌고 그의 몸 한쪽 면이 마비되었다.

23. 돌아가시다: 나는 그가 돌아가셨다는 소리를 듣고 깜짝 놀랐다.

24. 기절하다: 그녀는 머리를 부딪쳐서 기절했다.

나는 더위로 기절할 뻔 했다.

25. 소아의사: 그는 소아과의사에게 그의 아들의 죽음에 대하여 질문했다.

Ms. Smith는 소아과 전문의다.

26. 사라지다: 삼백 명의 사람들이 지진으로 사라졌다.

27. 약국: 24시간 여는 약국이 근처에 있나요?

28. 육체적인: 그녀는 외모에 집착한다.

29. 내과의사: 나는 전문임상간호사이고 나의 남편은 내과의사이다.

30. 알약: 나의 어머니는 하루에 알약을 세 번 또는 네 번 먹는다.

31. 성형수술: 그녀는 코를 성형수술 했다.

32. 처방하다: 이 약은 종종 우울증에 처방된다.

33. 맥박: 그녀의 맥박은 매우 약하다.

34. 회복하다: 수술로부터 회복되는 데 오랜 시간이 걸렸다.

경찰은 도난당한 물품의 일부분만 찾았다.

35. 재활치료하다: 알코올 중독자들을 재활시키는 특수 시설이 있어요.

36. 치료하다: 우리는 이 상황을 치료하기 위해서 재빠르게 행동해야 한다.

37. 타액: 타액은 충치를 예방하는 데 있어서 중요한 역할을 한다.

38. 모양: "어떻게 지내니?" "아주 건강해, 고마워"

39. 부작용: 이 약은 어떤 부작용이 있나요?

40. 뱉어내다, 침: 그는 구역질로 고기를 뱉어냈다.

선생님은 침을 많이 튀긴다. 그녀는 침으로 뒤범벅되어 있는 아기의 얼굴을 닦았다.

41. 접질림(삠): 너의 발목이 접질리거나 삐였을 동안에, 상처 입은 몸의 일부분이 쉴 수 있도록 잘 돌보아야 한다.

42. 청진기: 저에게 청진기를 건네줄 수 있겠습니까?

43. 고통을 겪다: 그녀는 몇 년 동안 암으로 고통을 받았다.

44. 질식사하다: 경찰 보고서에 따르면 희생자들이 연기에 질식사 했다고 말했다.

45. 외과의사: 외과의사는 너의 복부절개를 통해 복강경을 통과시켰다.

46. 수술: 그 환자는 뇌수술을 했다.

47. 붓다: 그의 뒤틀린 발목이 붓기 시작했다.

48. 치료: 그는 처방된 물리치료를 두 번 했다.

49. 충치: 충치는 세계에서 가장 흔한 건강질병 중 하나이다.

50. 수혈: 그녀의 목숨을 구하려면 수혈이 필요합니다.

51. 운송하다: 많은 질병은 오염된 물을 통해서 감염된다.

52. 이식: 그는 신장이식을 기다리는 중이다.

53. 치료: 희생자들은 응급구조원에 의해 응급처치를 받았다.

　　　그는 암 치료를 받고 있는 중이다.

54. 백신: 이 예방접종은 독감 바이러스로부터 보호한다.

55. 입원실: 입원실에 많은 환자들이 있다.

　　　모기를 퇴치하기 위해서 방충제를 사용해라.

56. 상처: 그의 상처가 치료되는데 몇 주가 걸렸다.

03. 질병 및 증상을 나타내는 단어

1. 급성의: 우리는 더 나은 연료사용을 통해서 만성과 급성의 호흡기 질환감염을 예방 할 수 있다.

2. 치매: 말기 치매환자들은 일반적으로 침대에 누워있고 의사소통이 불가능하다.

3. 기억상실증: 그녀는 노년에 기억상실을 겪었다.

4. 빈혈: 빈혈은 피곤함과 창백함을 초래할 수 있다.

5. 거식증: 거식증과 같은 섭식장애는 증가하고 있다.

6. 관절염: 관절염을 겪고 있는 몇 명의 아이들은 낮은 식욕을 가지고 있다.

7. 천식: 심각한 천식발작은 호흡이 멈추거나 죽음을 초래할 수 있다.

8. 조류독감: 조류독감 바이러스는 닭이나 야생 조류를 비롯해 새들을 감염시킨다.

9. 물집: 나는 주말에 발에 화상을 입었는데 물집이 잡히기 시작했다.

　　　그들은 엄청난 더위 속에 밖으로 나갔다.

10. 충혈: 수면부족으로 그녀의 눈은 충혈되었다.

11. 코피: 코피를 멈출 수 있는 법을 알려 줄래?

12. 폭식증: Wales의 공주는 20대 내내 폭식증으로부터 고통을 겪었다고 보고된다.

13. 암: 그는 작년에 간암으로 죽었다.

14. 수두: 수두는 어린이들 사이에서 흔한 질병이다.

15. 콜레라: 콜레라는 장 기관에 영향을 끼치는 세균질환이다.

16. 만성의: 그는 만성 우울증으로 고통을 겪었다.

17. 감기, 차갑다, 추운: 그녀는 감기에 걸렸다. 나의 발은 차갑다. 오늘은 얼듯이 춥다.

18. 변비: 사람뿐만 아니라 동물들도 변비로 고생을 한.

　　더 많은 식이섬유를 소비하면 너는 변비에 걸리지 않을 것이다.

19. 기침: 기침이나 재채기를 할 때 입을 가리고 해라.

20. 당뇨병: 약 1,700만 명의 미국인들이 당뇨병을 앓고 있고 그 숫자는 매년 증가하고 있다.

21. 설사: 비만방지 약은 지방흡수를 막는다. 그러나 가스나 설사 같은 부작용을 유발할 수 있다.

22. 어지러운: 나는 쉽게 가쁜 숨과 어지러움을 느낀다.

23. 졸리다: 나는 감기약을 먹는데, 그것은 나를 졸리게 만든다.

24. 귀통: 나는 귀통(이통)이 있다.

25. 열: 그는 두통과 약간의 열이 있다.

　　일본문화의 열풍은 1990년대에 아시아를 강타했다.

26. 심장발작: John은 3년 전에 심장발작을 일으켰다.

27. 고혈압: 고혈압일 때 동맥 내의 혈압은 증가한다.

28. 불면증: Holly는 그녀 어머니의 죽음 이후에 몇 달 동안 불면증에 시달렸다.

29. 가려운: 그 스웨터를 입으니 온몸이 가렵다.

　　나는 울을 입지 못한다. 왜냐하면 너무 가렵기 때문이다.

　　나는 일본에 가고 싶어 몸이 근질거릴 지경이다.

30. 나병: 나병은 인간의 역사가 시작된 이래로 무서운 질병이었다.

31. 백혈병: 모유 수유하는 아기들은 백혈병 발병의 위험이 더 낮다.

32. 광우병: 광우병 발병에 따라서 돼지고기 수요가 증가했다.

33. 홍역: 홍역은 전형적인 피부발진으로 잘 알려져 있다.

34. 멀미: 생강은 멀미를 예방하는데 도움이 된다.

35. 매스꺼움: 나는 생선회를 먹은 후에 매스꺼움을 느꼈다.

   그 약은 생각만 해도 매스꺼움을 느끼게 한다.

36. 창백한: 너는 창백해 보인다.

37. 폐렴: 감기가 악화되어서 폐렴으로 전이되었다.

38. 콧물: 나는 오늘 콧물이 난다.

39. 재채기: 나는 고양이 때문에 재채기를 한다. 내가 추측하기에 고양이 털 알레르기가 있는 것 같다.

40. 코골다: 그 남자가 너무 시끄럽게 코를 골아서 밤새 잠을 잘 수가 없어.

   나는 그의 끔찍한 코골이 소리에 참을 수 없다.

41. 아픈: 먼지 입자들에 눈이 아프다.

   이것이 네 눈에 거슬리니?

42. 무게, 부담, 균락: 너의 뼈는 너무 약해서 갑작스런 무게에 골절을 초래할 수 있다.

   초과된 몸무게는 너의 심장에 많은 부담을 준다.

   새롭고 더 위험한 바이러스 변종이 발견되었다.

43. 뇌졸중: 뇌졸중은 의학적인 응급사태이고 신속한 뇌졸중 치료가 중요하다.

44. 막힘: 이 알약을 먹으면 코 막힘이 나아질지도 몰라.

45. 증상: 그녀는 HIV 증상진행이 시작되었다.

46. 말기: 그녀는 폐암 말기 진단을 받았다.

47. 토하다: 나는 토할 것 같다. 그는 아침에 토했다.

04. 기타 건강관련 단어

1. 통증: 나는 온몸이 쑤시고 아프다. 나는 몸살이다.

2. 눈이 멀다: 그녀는 60대부터 시력을 잃기 시작했다.

   나는 어제 첫 소개팅을 했다.

3. 쥐나다: 나는 갑자기 수영 중에 다리 쥐가 났다.

4. 귀가 멀다: 그는 태어났을 때부터 완전히 귀가 멀었다.

5. 지친: 나는 지쳤다.

6. 원시: 나는 너무 원시가 심해서 안경 없이는 신문을 읽을 수가 없다.

7. 절뚝거리다: Mario는 다리를 다쳐서 절뚝거리며 운동장을 떠났다.

그는 절뚝거리며 걸었다.

8. 조용한: 대통령은 그 프로젝트에 대해 침묵을 유지했다.

9. 낮잠: 할아버지는 점심 후 낮잠을 주무신다.

10. 감각이 없는: 나의 손가락은 추위로 감각이 없다.

나의 엉덩이는 어머니가 때려서 여전히 감각이 없다.

11. 긁다: Hannah는 모기 물린 곳을 긁었다.

2. Expression

01. 리셉션에서 도움이 되는 표현법

1. 무엇을 도와드릴까요?

2. 보험증이나 신분증이 있으신가요?

3. 얼마정도 여기 계실 생각이세요?(얼마나 오래 여기 머무시나요?)

4. 한국에선 무슨 일을 하고 계세요?

5. 누가 당신에게 저희 치과를 추천해 주셨나요?

6. 잠시만 기다려주시겠어요?

7. 즉시 도와드릴게요.

8. 의자에 앉아 보시겠어요.

9. 누워 보세요, 한 번 보겠습니다.

10. 예전에 심각하게 아프신 적 있었나요?

11. 당신의 머리를 뒤로 눕히세요.

12. 편안하십니까?

13. 긴장푸시고 편안하게 계세요.

02. 치과병력

1. 방문의 목적(이유)

2. 가장 최근(마지막)에 치과방문은 언제입니까?

3. 잇솔질은 얼마나 자주 하십니까?

4. 사용하시는 칫솔모가 어떻습니까?(부드러움/중모/강모)

5. 양치하는 동안 잇몸에 출혈이 있습니까?

6. 치실 사용시 잇몸에 출혈이 있습니까?

7. 양치할 때나 혹은 치실 사용 시 치아의 일부분에서 아픔을 느끼나요?

8. 당신의 치아가 뜨겁고 차갑고 달거나 신 음식/음료에 반응(민감)합니까?

9. 당신의 치아가 흔들린다고 느낀 적이 있나요?

10. 음식물이 치아사이에 끼는 경향이 있나요?

11. 당신의 구강 안이나 입 주위가 아프거나 혹 같은 것이 있다고 느끼나요?

12. 당신의 턱에 다음과 같은 문제를 경험해본 적 있나요?

    *딸깍거리는 소리가 남, 턱관절 이상

    *관절, 귀, 얼굴면의 통증

    *개폐구시의 어려움(입을 열고 다물 때)

    *교합시의 통증(씹을 때)

13. 당신은 머리나 목, 턱에 상처가 있습니까?

14. 당신은 두통을 자주 경험하십니까?

15. 깨어있거나 수면 중에 당신은 치아를 깨물거나 갈기도 합니까?

16. 당신은 입술이나 뺨을 자주 깨뭅니까?

17. *교정치료 받으신 적 있습니까?

    *구강수술 받으신 적 있습니까?

    *치은(치주)치료 받으신 적 있습니까?

    *당신은 교합조정 받으신 적 있습니까?

    *소아치과교정을 받으신 적 있습니까?

18. 당신의 치아외형에 만족하십니까?

19. 당신은 치과에서 언짢은 경험을 해보신 적 있습니까?

20. 치과치료가 당신을 괴롭게 했던 점이 있습니까?

03. 통증에 관한 표현법

1. 어떻게 오셨습니까?

2. 통증이 있으십니까?

3. 어제보다는 좀 나아지신 것 같으세요?

4. 어디가 아프세요?

5. 당신의 증상을 설명해 주시겠습니까?

6. 어느 종류의 통증입니까?

7. 얼마나 자주 통증을 느끼십니까?

8. 우둔하게 아프십니까?

9. 날카롭게 아프십니까?

10. 욱씬거리는 통증입니까?

11. 계속적으로 아프신지요?

12. 가끔씩 아프신지요?

13. 칼로 찌르는 통증입니까?

14. 지속적으로 아프신가요?

15. 입을 다물 때 아프신가요?

16. 이 치아를 두드릴 때 아프신가요?

17. 단음식이나 차갑고 따뜻한 온도나 직접적인 접촉에 예민하신가요?

18. 뜨거우십니까? (차가우십니까?)

19. 씹으실 때 어떠세요?

20. 이제 제가 체크해보겠습니다.

21. 제가 건드렸을 때 아프신가요?

22. 이런 증상이 얼마나 오래되었습니까?

23. 얼마나 오래 지속되고 있습니까?

24. 제가 한번 보겠습니다.

25. 아프시면 말씀하세요.

26. 그리 심각한 것은 아닙니다.

27. 심각하지는 않은 것 같습니다.

04. 수술 후에 표현법

1. 머리를 뒤로 하세요.

2. 머리를 오른쪽으로 돌리세요.

3. 입을 약간 다물어보세요.

4. 할 수 있는 한 크게 입을 벌려보세요.

5. 편안하세요?

6. 긴장푸시고 편안하게 계세요.

7. 내일 다시 오실 수 있으세요?

8. 기다리게 해서 죄송합니다.

9. 월요일 오후에 오실 수 있으신가요?

10. 오전중이나 오후, 어느 시간이 더 편하신가요?

11. 당신 회복이 잘 되어서 기쁩니다.

12. 붓거나 아프시면 연락해주세요.

13. 입안에 있는 이물질을 행구어 내세요.

14. 내일까지 양치하지 마세요.

15. 피가 얼마동안 났었습니까?(출혈이 얼마나 지속됐습니까?)

16. 지금은 아프지 않으시죠? 그렇죠?

17. 조심하시고, 곧 괜찮아질 겁니다.

18. 열이 계속되시면 알려주세요.

19. 유동식을 많이 드시고, 말을 많이 하는 걸 피해주세요.

20. 입맛은 어떠세요?

21. 통증을 줄이기 위해 주사와 약을 드리겠습니다.

22. 며칠 후에 다시 뵙겠습니다.

05. 방사선에 도움이 되는 표현법

1. 진단을 하기위해서 방사선촬영(진단)이 필요합니다.

2. 방사선촬영은 구강 내의 상태를 정확하게 보여줄 것입니다.

3. 저를 따라오세요.

4. 지금 저와 방사선촬영실로 같이 가실게요.

5. 방사선촬영을 하겠습니다.

6. 언제 마지막으로 방사선촬영을 하셨나요?

7. 임산부이신가요?

8. 임신 가능성이 있으신가요?

9. 손가락으로 필름을 잡아 주세요.

10. 엄지손가락으로 그것을 잡아주세요.

11. 안경을 벗어주길 바랍니다.

12. 여기 서 주시고, 판 위에 턱을 놓아주세요.

13. 손으로 손잡이를 잡아주세요.

14. 움직이지 마세요!

15. 방사선사진을 현상하는데 5분 정도 소요됩니다. (순서체크 필요)

16. '삐' 소리가 날 때까지 움직이지 마세요.

17. 협조해 주셔서 감사합니다.

18. 이쪽으로 오십시오.

19. 방사선필름을 현상할 때까지 2~3분정도 기다려주시기 바랍니다.

20. 필름이 곧 현상될 것입니다.

21. 방사선이 현상된 후 설명을 드릴게요.

22. 의사선생님께서 더 자세하게 방사선사진에 대해 설명을 드릴 것입니다.

23. 방사선에서 특별한 소견이 보이지 않습니다.

3. Reading Comprehension

01. 구강위생과 치과질환

　대부분의 사람들은 주요한 신체구조 중에 한부분인 치아를 가지고 있고, 또한 치아는 음식을 저작하는 주요한 기능을 하며, 그것은 음식을 삼키게 해준다. 치아는 구강 내에서 음식을 자르고 씹을 수 있게 해주는 하얗고 딱딱한 주체이다. 사람들은 무언가를 항상 먹어야만 하며 사회에서 많은 동료들과 이야기를 해야만 한다.

　구강은 혀, 타액, 치아 입술로 구성되어 있다. 사람들은 먹어야만 하고 그 구강은 타액으로 젖어있기 때문에 구강위생이 아주 중요하다. 따라서 구강위생은 구강이 잘 유지될 수 있도록 습관되어야 하며, 치아우식과 치주질환을 예방해야 한다.

　만약 사람들이 구강관리를 소홀히 한다면, 치태 및 세균, 구취가 있을 수 도 모른다. 또한 최악의 경우는 치아상실을 초래할지도 모른다. 게다가 치아가 없는 사람들은 나이든 사람으로 보일 수도 있고 음식을 씹는데 어려워 그 결과 소화를 어렵게 할 수도 있다.

　이러한 이유로, 구강위생은 모든 사람들이 건강한 치아와 구강을 유지할 수 있도록 반드시 필요하다.

02. 치아우식과 치주질환의 비교

　보고서에서는 치아우식과 치주질환이 양대 구강병이라고 설명하고 있다. 치아우식은 어린이들에게 있어 치아상실을 야기시킬 수 있는 질병이며, 반면에 치주질환은 성인 사이에 치아상실이 되는 질병이다.

A. 치아우식

　치과에서 이 질병은 충지 및 치아파괴, 치아손상의 원인 되어 치아에 구멍이 생긴 것을 의미한다. 치아우식은 사탕이나 단음식을 즐겨먹는 미취학 어린이들이 치아를 잘 돌보지 않는데서 원인된다. 따라서 치아우식으로부터 예방하기 위해 스스로의 치아관리를 잘 해야만 한다.

B. 치주질환

치주질환은 잇몸질환이다. 치주질환은 건강한 잇몸과 치조골을 가지고 있지 않는 35세 이상의 성인집단에서 발생한다. 치주관리는 치아의 구조를 지지해주기 때문에 중요하다. 치주질환은 잇몸과 치아주위에 치태나 치석이 둘러 싸여 잇몸에 피가 스며나오는 것이 주된 현상이다.

치료되지 않은 치주질환의 과정: 부착치은이 치근단 쪽으로 향해서 퇴축되며, 그 뒤 그 치아는 점차적으로 흔들리게 되며 결국 치아가 빠지게 되는 것이다.

03. 신경치료

신경치료는 좀 더 정확히 이야기 하자면 근관치료이며 치과에서 널리 알려져 있는 전문분야중 하나이다. 치아의 내측면에 신경이 있다는 것으로 알려져 있다. 그것은 신경관과 혈관으로 구성되어져 있다. 어금니는 주로 치근이 하나 이상 있는데 각 치근마다 한 개 또는 두 개 이상의 신경관이 있다.

이 신경은 주로 치아의 외형에 의해 보호받고 있다. 충치가 생겼거나 금이 치아 보호벽을 파괴했을 때, 그 신경은 구강 내 세균에 노출된다. 이것은 염증, 감염 점차적으로 농양의 결과로 초래할 수 있다.

근관치료는 전이된 신경을 제거해줄 뿐만 아니라 그 치아를 건강한 상태로 돌려준다. 또한 치아로부터 감염된 모든 것을 제거해준다. 이 치료는 치과선생님께서 환자에게 마취주사를 주기 때문에 그다지 아프지 않을 것이다. 그리고 어떤 시술을 하기 전에 그 치아가 감각이 없는지를 확실히 해야만 한다.

신경치료가 마무리될 때, 신경치료 그 자체의 성공뿐만 아니라 그 치아기능을 완전히 복원시키는 것이 중요하다. 대부분의 어금니는 금관이나 완전 수복 보철을 해야 한다.

현대의 의학기술과 진통제로, 대부분의 사람들이 충치로 가득찬 부분만큼 근관충전으로 채우는 것은 주목할 만한 것이 아니라고 보고한다. 치료 후에 처방전 없이 살 수 있는 진통제는 느끼고 있는 어떤 위안을 경감시켜준다.

근관치료는 높은 성공률을 자랑하고 인간의 몸 자체가 완전하게 치료할 수 있는 보장은 없다는 것이다. 이러한 이유로, 치료가 다 끝난 후에라도 정기 검진을 받기 위해 치과에 가야 하는 것이 중요하다.

환자의 이해와 협조가 신경치료의 한 부분으로서 아주 중요하다.

04. 건강한 치아를위한 TBI와 식이조절

치과위생사들은 치아건강을 위해 TBI와 식이조절에 대해서 제안한다.

첫 번째 적어도 하루에 세 번, 음식을 먹은 후 3분 이내에 3분 동안 규칙적으로 충치를 없애기 위해 치아를 닦아야 한다. 일반적으로 칫솔은 짧은 머리와 편평한 모와 구부림이 없는 손잡이를 가져야 한다. 또한 칫솔은 완전히 말린 후에 사용해야 한다. 칫솔은 감기와 독감 같은 병이 걸린 이후, 또는 2~3개월 마다 교체해야 한다.

두 번째, 식이조절은 중요하다. 왜냐하면 사람들은 보통 다양한 음식을 먹는다. 이러한 이유로 사람들은 모든 설탕이 든 음식을 줄여야 한다. 왜냐하면 이런 음식은 충치를 유발한다. 치과위생을 위한 치아건강은 과일과 채소이다. 또한 샐러드와 당근 또한 사과를 먹는 것은 음식 찌꺼기가 빠져나갈 수 있게 도와준다.

내가 뭘 먹어야 하는가?

전체적 건강과 구강건강을 위한 충분한 영양섭취를 확실히 하기위해서는 당신은 매일마다 다음에 나오는 기본 음식 그룹에서 몇몇 음식들을 선택해야만 한다.

- 식빵, 시리얼, 밥과 파스타
- 야채
- 과일
- 우유, 요거트와 치즈
- 고기, 새고기, 생선, 말린 콩, 달걀과 넛츠
- 지방, 기름과 달콤한 것들 - 적게 사용해라.

무슨 음식을 먹으면 안 되는가?

당신은 음식을 먹을 때 스낵, 부드러운 것을 피하고 달콤하고 끈적끈적한 음식, 케이크, 사탕, 말린 과일과 같은 음식은 치아에 달라붙기에 치아우식을 촉진한다.

대신에 구강에 좋은 음식은 견과류와 생채소와 같은 플레인 요거트와 치즈와 팝콘과 무설탕 껌과 사탕을 선택해라.

어떤 솔을 사용해야 하는가?

식사 후와 간식을 먹은 후에 칫솔질 하는 것은 음식의 작은 입자뿐만이 제거되는 것이 아니라 치태와 끈쩍한 덩어리를 제거한다. 치태는 산을 제공하는 박테리아에 의해 만들어지고 치아우식과 잇몸질환을 유발하고 칫솔질하는 주요 목표는 치태를 철저히 제거하는 것이다.

불소치약을 사용하는 것은 박테리아 정도를 감소하고 또한 치아표면을 재광화시키고 그들을 더 강하게 만드는데 중요하다.

당신은 치과의사 또는 치과위생사는 당신을 위해서 최고의 칫솔을 추천해준다. 일반적으로 부드러운 솔과 끝이 둥글거나 윤기가 있는 모는 잇몸조직 상처 또는 치아표면 손상을 덜 줄 수 있다.

칫솔의 크기나 모양과 각은 각각 치아에 도달할 수 있도록 해야 한다. 어린이들은 성인을 위한 것 보다 칫솔이 더 작은 것이 필요하다.

기억해라: 닳은 칫솔은 치아를 적절히 깨끗하게 해주지 못하며, 잇몸에 상처를 줄 것이다.

칫솔은 3~4개월마다 교체해야한다.

치과의 비상사태

입에 관한 손상은 뽑은 치아, 돌출된 이, 관절된 이를 포함한다.

때때로 입술, 잇몸, 턱은 다치기도 한다. 입 관련 손상은 흔히 아프고 가능한 빠른 시일내에 치과의사의 진료를 받아야 한다.

치아가 빠졌을 때 당신이 해야만 할 것

- 치아를 찾기 위해 노력하라.
- 긴급 상황에 즉시 치과의사를 불러라.
- 부드럽게 헹구고 치아에 있는 이물질 제거를 위해 너무 쌔게 문지르지 마라.
- 잇몸과 턱 사이에 깨끗한 치아를 놓아라.
- 소켓 안에 다시 치아를 놓지 마라. 이것은 더 큰 손상을 줄 수가 있다.
- 가능한 빨리 치과의사한테 가라. 만약 손상된지 삼십분을 넘지 않는다면 다시 치아를 심을 수 있다.
- 만약 외상이 심한 사람의 입안에 빠진 치아를 보관 할 수 없다면(예를 들면, 어린아이의 경우) 깨끗한 천이나 거즈에 싸서 우유에 담궈라.

05. 맹출하는 사랑니는 충치나 잇몸질환을 진행시킬지도 모른다.

주로 사람의 턱은 새 어금니가 맹출할 때 지지해 줄 수 있는 여유가 충분하지 않다. 그 치아는 잇몸을 뚫고 못 올라올 수도 있고 대신에 턱 안쪽으로 매복되어 있을 수도 있다. 맹출 하는 치아는 다른 치아에 겹쳐서 올라올 수 있는 가능성도 있고, 통증도 있으며 감염 또는 염증, 잇몸을 붓게 한다.

맹출 중인 사랑니는 충치나 잇몸질환을 진행시킬지도 모르다. 왜냐하면 그 치아는 깨끗하게 하기가 어렵기 때문이다. 사랑니의 대부분의 문제는 15~25세 사이에 진행된다.

30세 이상에서 문제를 야기 시키는 소수의 사람들은 사랑니 발치가 요구되어진다. 대부분의 치과 선생님은 16~19세 사이의 사람들에게 사랑니가 맹출한다는 것을 알고 있다. 대부분의 치과선생님은 말썽이 되는 사랑니를 제거하기 위해 20세까지 기다리지 말라고 충고한다. 왜냐하면 치아주위의 턱이 계속적으로 성장하고 딱딱하기 때문이다. 발치는 더욱 어렵고 어른들에 있어서 치유는 느려진다는 것이다.

09. What do you know about healthcare?

④ Reading

A. 우리는 보통 두통, 치통, 복통 등과 같은 것들을 완화시키기 위해서 진통제를 사용합니다. 이것을 한번 상상해봅시다. 어금니에 있는 당신 치아 중에 하나가 정말로 아픕니다. 당신은 치과의사에게 진찰을 받아야한다고 생각하지만, 치과의사에게 가는 것을 몹시 무서워합니다. 당신은 진통제를 먹습니다. 당신은 훨씬 안도하며, 일상생활을 계속 유지할 수 있습니다. 이제, 당신이 치통을 느낄 때 마다, 의사에게 진찰을 받는 것 대신에 진통제를 먹습니다. 이것은 쉬운 방법일 수도 있으나, 심각한 문제를 일으킬 수도 있습니다. 당신의 질환이 좀 더 나빠질 수도 있고, 불쾌한 부작용을 경험할 수도 있습니다. 그러므로, 진통제는 꼭 필요할 경우에만 처방전과 함께 사용되어야 합니다. 그리고 지시사항을 올바르게 따라야 합니다.

B. 대부분의 상처는 보통 가볍고, 대부분의 가벼운 상처는 몇 분 안에 피가 멈춥니다. 그래서 그것들은 집에서 쉽게 치료할 수 있습니다. 첫 번째, 상처 안의 먼지를 제거하고 차가운 물과 함께 상처를 씻습니다. 이렇게 함으로써, 당신은 감염의 위험을 없앨 수 있습니다. 당신은 비누를 사용해서는 안됩니다. 그뒤 상처부위를 건조시키고 항생연고를 바르거나 붕대를 감으면 됩니다. 붕대를 종종 교체함으로써 깨끗한 붕대를 사용해야 합니다. 그러나, 상처가 좀 더 심각하고 아주 깊다면, 당신은 즉시 병원에 가야 합니다. 상처를 꿰매야 하거나 추가적인 치료를 요할지도 모릅니다.

C. 홍역 발생이 있으며 많은 사람들이 홍역에 걸리고 있습니다. 만약 당신이 홍역에 걸린다면, 당신이 인지해야 할 첫 번째 증상은 목 주위의 피부발진입니다. 다른 증상들로는 콧물, 복통 그리고 기침을 포함합니다. 피로를 느낄 수 있으며, 음식섭취와 수면에 문제가 생길 수 있습니다. 이러한 증상들은 약 7일 정도 지속될 것입니다. 치료방법은 없으나, 의사가 당신들에게 도움이 되는 약을 처방해 줄 수 있습니다. 홍역은 보통 심각하진 않고, 자연스럽게 낫습니다. 그러나 몇몇 사람들에겐 홍역증상이 심각해 질 수 있으므로, 이러한 증상들 중 하나를 알게 된다면 당신은 의사에게 진찰을 받아야 합니다.

D. 당신의 건강상태가 좋을 때 건강검진을 받는 것이 시간낭비일 것 같다는 것을 잘 알고 있습니다. 그러나 건강검진을 위해 병원에 가는 것은 큰 병이 생기기전에 건강상의 작은 문제를 찾는 중요한 방법입니다. 예를 들어, 심전도검사는 큰 문제가 되기 전에 심장관련 질환들을 찾아 낼 수 있습니다. 우리들 대부분은 직장이나 학업 때문에 너무 바빠서 일상적 생활건강에 대해서 관심을 갖지 못합니다. 우리는 종종 충분한 수면을 취하지 못하고 패스트푸드를 섭취합니다. 우리의 현대생활습관은 건강상의 문제를 일으킬 수 있습니다. 정기적으로 병원에 가는 것은 당신이 건강을 유지하는데 도움이 될 수 있습니다.

E. 주립대학에서, 우리의 간호학위는 완전하게 승인된 4년제 대학과정입니다. 교육과정의 처음 2년동안에는, 화학, 생물학, 그리고 생리학과 같은 기초과정을 들을 것입니다. 처음 2년의 과정을 마친 후에는, 당신은 간호사로서의 실습과정을 시작할 것입니다. 마지막 2년동안, 당신은 대부분의 시간을 실제환자들과 함께 병원에서 일을 하며 시간을 보낼 것입니다. 당신은 또한 의사들의 감독하에 일을 하게 될 것입니다. 실습과정의 마지막 해에는, 당신은 환자들에게 주사를 놓을 수 있고, 의사들이 환자를 치료할 때 그들을 보조할 수 있을 것입니다. 실습기간동안에 저는 심지어 부러진 팔에 깁스하는 것과 같은 일도 할 수 있었습니다. 정말 흥미로웠습니다.

F. 비록 여러분이 매 식사 후에 이를 닦고 규칙적으로 여러분의 치아에 치실을 이용할지라도, 적어도 1년에 두 번은 치과에 가야합니다. 여러분이 치과에 가는 것은, 스스로가 몇몇 치아문제들을 예방하는 것입니다. 물론, 치과에 가는 것이 여러분 치아를 보호하는 것입니다. 치과의사는 충치를 치료하기 쉬울 때, 그와 같은 문제들을 탐지할 수 있습니다. 사람들이 나이가 들어감에 따라, 치은염/치주염은 치아상실의 가장 흔한 이유가 됩니다. 치과의사는 치은염의 초기증상을 파악하여 그것을 치료할 수 있습니다. 의사들은 또한 암과 같은 심각한 질환을 검진할 수 있습니다. 구강암은 세상에서 6번째로 흔한 암 형태입니다. 암으로부터 살아남는 방법은 조기진단이므로, 치과검진을 자주 하시길 바랍니다.

4. Dialogue

01 Dental English

① Dialogue 1

Sam **S**   Receptionist **R**

S 안녕하세요. 10시 30분에 피터슨 선생님께 예약 약속을 했습니다.

R 안녕하세요. 성함을 여쭤봐도 될까요?

S 네. 샘 워터스입니다

R 네 워터스씨. 피터슨 선생님께 진료받는게 처음이에요?

S 아니요, 보험카드가 변경되었습니다. 여기 새로운 카드가 있습니다.

R 감사합니다. 오늘 치과선생님께서 특별히 치료할 부분이 있나요?

S 네. 최근에 잇몸이 아파요.

R 알겠습니다. 기록해 두겠습니다.

S 그리고, 치아뿐만 아니라 스켈링도 하고 싶습니다.

R 물론, 워터스씨는 오늘 구강관리의 한 부분이 될 것입니다.

S 아~~네 좋아요.

R 네 의자에 앉아주세요. 의사 피터슨 선생님께서 곧 오실 것입니다.

S 고맙습니다.

R 천만에요.

② Dialogue 2

Sam ⑤   Dr. peterson ⓓ

⑤ 안녕하세요? 의사선생님

ⓓ 안녕하세요. 샘, 오늘 하루 어때요?

⑤ 저는 좋습니다!! 최근에 잇몸이 조금 아파요.

ⓓ 음. . . 한번 살펴보겠습니다. 뒤로 기대시고 입을 벌려주세요. 네 아주 좋아요.

⑤ (검진 후) 어때요?

ⓓ 음 . . 잇몸일부에 염증이 있습니다. 제 생각으로는 x-ray를 찍어야 될 것 같아요.

⑤ 네? 무슨 말이에요? 많이 심각하나요?

ⓓ 아니요. 매년 하는 일반적인 진행 절차입니다. 아마 몇 개의 충치가 있는 걸로 보이네요.

⑤ 좋은 소식은 아니네요.

ⓓ 두 개 정도 충치가 있는 것 같으며 그것들은 표면에 있는 것 같아요.

⑤ 저도 그러기를 바래요.

ⓓ 우리는 충치의 진행 정도를 알아보기 위해 x-ray를 찍고 마찬가지로 치아사이에 충치가 더 있는지 점검
   해야 할 필요가 있어요.

⑤ 알겠어요.

ⓓ 여기 방사선용 에이프런을 입어주세요.

⑤ 알겠습니다.
   (방사선 촬영 후)

ⓓ X-ray를 찍어 보니 진행 중인 충치는 더 이상 없는 것 같아요.

⑤ 좋은 소식이네요.

ⓓ 네. 치아 2개만 와동충전하고 스켈링을 하시면 됩니다.

③ Dialogue 3

Sam **S**   Gina the dental hygienist **G**

S 안녕하세요?

G 안녕하세요. 워터스씨 저는 치과위생사 지나입니다. 오늘 스켈링을 해드리겠습니다.

S 피터슨씨는 충치 2개 치료해주셨습니다. 왜 스켈링을 해야 하나요?

G 저희는 워터스씨의 치아와 잇몸을 깨끗하게 해드리고 질병에 이환되지 않게 건강한
상태로 해드리려고 합니다.

S 이제 이해가 되네요.

G 구강건강은 치아 문제가 생기지 않도록 해줍니다. 플라그제거를 시작할게요.
입을 벌려주세요.

S 네, 안 아프게 해주세요.

G 비록 모든 사람들이 정기적으로 치실 사용을 하더라도 플라그가 있습니다.
검진을 위해 일 년에 두 번씩 치과에 와야 할 중요한 이유입니다.
(스케링을 하는 중 말을 잘 하지 못함)
물을 마시고 입을 헹구세요.

S 오~~한결 나아졌군요.

G 지금은 불소도포를 할 것입니다. 어떤 맛으로 해드릴까요?

S 제가 선택해요?

G 물론, 우리는 민트, 박하, 오렌지맛, 어린이들을 위한 풍선껌 맛이 있어요.

S 저는 풍선껌 맛으로 할래요!!

G 네, 지금 치실을 이용해 마무리 드리겠습니다.

Ⓢ 선생님 어떤 타입의 치실을 추천 해주시겠어요?

Ⓖ 저는 개인적으로 납작한 형태의 치실을 좋아합니다. 치아 사이에 더 잘 들어가기 때문입니다.

Ⓢ 네, 기억해두었다가 다음에 그 치실을 사야겠습니다. 얼마나 자주 치실을 사용하나요?

Ⓖ 매일요, 하루에 최소한 두 번씩, 일부 사람들은 식사하고 난 뒤에 매일 치실을 사용하지만 그것이 반드시 필요한 것은 아닙니다.

Ⓢ (스켈링을 다 끝내고 난 뒤) 너무 상쾌합니다. 감사합니다.

Ⓖ 천만에요. 매일 치실 사용 기억하시구요. 적어도 하루에 한 번은 하셔야 합니다.
그럼 즐거운 하루 되세요.

④ Dialogue 4

6개월마다 한 번씩 치석제거를 받아야 한다.

Doctor Ⓓ   Patient Ⓟ

Ⓓ 무슨 문제입니까, 마이클?

Ⓟ 내 입에 욱신거리는 통증이 있어요.

Ⓓ '아' 해보세요. 잇몸이 부어있네요.

Ⓟ 하지만 전 모르겠어요. 왜 두통까지 생기는지. . . . . .

Ⓓ 걱정마세요. 이것은 대부분 치통으로부터 오는 것입니다.

Ⓟ 음. . . . 2가지의 고통이 있어요. 그것은 엎친데 덮친격(설상가상)이네요.
제 구강상태가 심각한가요?

Ⓓ 그다지 심각하지 않은 것 같아요.

Ⓟ 그러면 수술이 필요하지 않나요?

Ⓓ X-ray검사 후에 더 자세하게 말씀 드리겠습니다.

Ⓟ 결과가 어떤가요?

Ⓓ 부은 잇몸은 심각하지 않습니다. 하지만 스켈링을 해야 합니다.

Ⓟ 스켈링이요?

Ⓓ 네, 잇몸이 부어있습니다. 왜냐하면 치석이 있기 때문입니다.

약간의 약을 처방해 드리겠습니다. 그러나 치석제거 하는 것을 잊지마세요.

6개월에 1번씩 스켈링을 받으셔야 합니다.

Ⓟ 네, 알겠습니다.

⑤ Dialogue 5

스켈링(치석제거를 해야 합니다)

RDH, Lee Ⓛ   Julia Ⓙ

Ⓛ 어떤가요? 저는 치위생사입니다. 제 이름은 Lee입니다.

Ⓙ 저는 아침에 당신의 이를 깨끗하게 해드릴 예정입니다.

Ⓛ 이전에 치석제거를 해 본 적이 있습니까?

Ⓙ 아니요, 전 태어나서 스켈링을 받아본 적이 한 번도 없습니다.

치아에 치석이 많이 있나요? 뭔가 잘못되었나요?

Ⓛ 당신의 입을 벌려주세요, 체크 먼저 하겠습니다.

하악 전치 뒤에 많은 침착물이 있습니다.

그리고, 유감스럽게도 당신은 양치질을 제대로 안한 것 같네요.

Ⓙ 어째서요? 매일 식사 후에 양치질을 했는데요.

Ⓛ 솔질로는 치석이 제거되지 않습니다.

당신은 치석제거를 6개월에 한 번씩 해야 합니다.

칫솔질 방법에 대해 설명해 줄 것이고, 치아를 깨끗이 한 후 칫솔질 교육법을 알려드리겠습니다.

편안히 계세요. 만약 통증을 느낀다면 손을 드세요.

치석제거를 할 때 고통을 느낄 수도 있고 잇몸주위에 출혈이 있을 수도 있습니다.

그렇지만, 걱정하지 마세요. 그다지 심각한 문제는 아닙니다.

Ⓙ 네, 알겠습니다. 편안히 있겠습니다.

Ⓛ (스켈링 후) 당신의 치아 표면을 매끄럽게 하겠습니다. 당신은 더 좋게 느낄 거예요.

Ⓙ 정말 감사합니다.

⑥ Dialogue 6

물속의 불소

Nancy Ⓝ   Alex Ⓐ

Ⓝ 안녕, 알렉스, 이번 주말에 뭐 했니?

Ⓐ 별로 신나는 일은 없었어. 화학과목 리포트를 써야 했어.

Ⓝ 아, 그렇구나. . . 뭐에 대해 썼는데

Ⓐ 불소화나트륨, 치약의 주요 성분이지. 수돗물에 그것을 첨가하는 나라도 많아.

Ⓝ 너무 따분한 내용 같다.

Ⓐ 들으면 의외겠지만, 사실은 굉장히 흥미롭고 논란이 많은 주제야.

N 그래? 왜 그런데?

A 음, 그게 독성이 강하거든. 만일 어린아이가 보통 크기의 치약 하나를 다 먹으면 죽을 정도로.

N 말도 안 돼! 그럼 치약 회사들은 왜 그걸 사용하는데?

A 아하! 거기에 불소의 비밀이 있어! 나도 정말 모르겠다니까. 공식적으로, 치약 회사들은 불소가 치아가 썩는 걸 막아준다고 주장해. 하지만, 레베카 칼리 같은 연구자들은 이걸 강력하게 반박하지. 그녀는 불소에 관한 연구는 조작되었고, 그 연구에 돈을 댄 회사들에 의해 연구원들이 부패했다고 주장해. 확실히, 그 연구의 실험 대상들은 충치가 적었는데, 그 이유는 불소를 오래 사용하다 결국 이가 빠져버렸기 때문이지!

N 끔찍하다! 마시는 수돗물에 불소를 넣는 것은 어때? 그것도 위험해?

A 음, 불소는 알루미늄 생산의 부산물이야. 알루미늄 생산업자들은 이 부산물을 합법적으로 처리하는데 드는 높은 비용을 감당하지 않으려고 이걸 수돗물 회사에 찾아. 그것은 큰 통에 넣어 팔리는데, 해골과 뼈가 교차된 그림이 붙어 있고 "독극물, 소량으로도 위험함!" 경고문이 그 통에 붙어있지. 그 화학물은 그런 다음에 급수 탱크에 버려져.

N 정말 황당하다! 내가 먹는 수돗물에는 불소가 들어 있지 않아야 할텐데.

A 미국, 캐나다, 오스트레일리아, 뉴질랜드 같은 대부분의 영어권 국가들을 수돗물 시스템에 불소를 넣어. 유럽 대륙 국가와 일본은 이미 그걸 금지했지만. 불소가 들어있는 다른 제품도 알고 있니?

N 아니... 몰라.

A 불소는 쥐약과 시중에서 파는 살충제, 특히 바퀴벌레 약에 들어 있어. 프로작 같은 항우울제에서도 중요한 성분이고, 칼리 박사는 불소가 독일 나치 수용소와 공산주의 러시아 수용소에서 처음으로 사용되었다고 주장하고 있어. 수감자들은 멍하게 만들어서 순종적으로 만들기 위해 사용한거지. 불소는 또한 일부 가공 식품과 음료수에도 들어 있어.

N 음, 불소에 대해 경고해 줘서 고마워. 지금부터는 조심해야겠다!.

⑦ Dialogue 7

Ms. Lee **L**   John's mom **M**

어린이들의 치아는 치아가 맹출 되는 시기에 잇솔질이 필요하다. (약 6개월경)

비록 어린이들이 스스로 잇솔질을 할수 있도록 권장해야만 하지만, 어린이들은 여섯살이 될때까지 스스로 즐겁게 철두철미하게 잇솔질을 할 수 없다. 그러므로 부모는 자식이 잇솔질을 끝낸후에 다시 한번 더 잇솔질을 해줘야 한다. 6살에서 12살 사이의 어린이들은 사진의 잇솔질 할 수 있는 능력이 될 수 있을 것이다.

그러나, 부모는 자식이 제대로 하고 있는지 보기 위해 정기적으로 체크를 해야만 한다. 이와 같은 같은 충고는 치실사용에도 적용된다. 그러나 대부분의 어린이들은 12살이 될때까지 적절하기 치실을 다룰수 가 없다. 그러므로 이것은 부모들의 책임을 져야만 한다.

존의 엄마는 자식의 치아를 어떻게 관리해야 하는지 배운다.

L 존과 엄마에게 잇솔질은 어떻게 하는지 보여드리겠습니다. 자, 존이 매일마다 잇솔질을 하게 하는 것은 엄마의 책임입니다.

M 행동을 하는 것보다 말로는 쉽습니다. 존이 잠자리에 들기 전에 '잇솔질해' 라고 말할 때 마다 항상 저를 속상하게 합니다.

L 존은 지쳐합니다. 엄마는 좀더 이른 낮 시간에 존의 잇솔질을 해야 할 것입니다.

M 그것 좋은 생각이네요

L 존이 여섯살이 될 때까지 적절하게 스스로 잇솔질을 할 수 없기 때문에 본인이 잇솔질을 하고 난 뒤에도 한번 더 잇솔질을 해주어야만 합니다.

M 그럼 훨씬 잘 되겠네요

ⓛ 네 맞습니다. 반드시 필요합니다. 그리고 하루에 최소한 한번은 치실 사용을 잊어버리지 마세요. 존은 10살 또는 12살이 될때까지 스스로 철저하게 치실 사용을 할 수 없을 것입니다.

Ⓜ 치실 사용법을 알려 주시겠어요?

ⓛ 쉽습니다. 첫번째 18인치 정도 치실을 준비합니다. 여기처럼 치실을 세번째 손가락에 감습니다. 여기요 (치과위생사는 치실을 엄마에게 건내준다) 함 해보세요.

Ⓜ 감사합니다.

ⓛ 자, 이와 같이 두번째 손가락과 엄지손가락을 이용해 치실을 움직여 보세요.

Ⓜ 쉽네요

ⓛ 구강내 두번째 손가락을 가죠. 대고 이와 같이 한쪽 방향만요.

Ⓜ 알겠습니다.

ⓛ 이제 치실을 치아사이에서 플라그가 제거될 수 있도록 열 번 정도 위아래로 올렸다 내렸다 해보세요.

Ⓜ 오케이. 지지~~ 치실이 이렇게 더러워 질 수가.

ⓛ 네 맞습니다. 치아 사이에 플라그가 많습니다.

Ⓜ 존의 치아를 위해서 어떻게 관리하는지 보여주셔서 감사합니다.

ⓛ 천만에요. 저의 일입니다.

02. Which doctor should I go to?

② Let's read

A. Reading Practice 1

Tina 🌓   Joey 🌘

🌓 헤이, Joey. 어제 어딨었니? 학교에서 못 봤는걸.

🌘 어, Tina야. 나 시력검사하러 갔었어. / 검안사 만나러 갔었어.

🌓 왜?

🌘 최근에 사물들을 볼 때 좀 문제가 있었어. 교실에서는 칠판이 항상 흐릿하고, 야구를 할 땐 투수를 잘 볼 수가 없어.

🌓 오, 이런. 검안사는 뭐라고 했니?

🌘 의사가 말하길, 내가 근시안이라서 안경을 써야 한다고 말했어

🌓 근시안이라는게, 네가 멀리있는 사물을 못 본다는 말 맞지?

🌘 정확해. 오늘 학교마치고 안경을 좀 고르러 갈거야. 좋은 안경 고르는 것 좀 도와주지 않을래? 다른 사람의 생각을 듣는 건 좋은 것 같아. 그러면 내가 제일 좋아 보이는 걸 고를 수 있으니깐. 어머니께서 말씀하시길, 제일 비싸고 유행하는 것이라도, 내가 갖고 싶은 안경 아무거나 사도 된다고 하셨어.

🌓 물론. 재밌을 것 같은데. 수업 마치고 정문에서 보자.

🌘 좋아, 근데 너 정확히 언제 올 수 있을 것 같니?

🌓 음... 3시 40분에 만나자. 괜찮니?

🌘 완전 좋아. 그 때 봐!

B. Reading Practice 2

❶ Dermatologist는 피부과 전문의이다. Dermatologists는 피부에 문제가 있는 사람들을 도와주며 다양한 피부질병을 치료할 수 있다. 사람들이 화상을 입거나 여드름과 같은 문제가 있을 때, dermatologist을 찾는다.

❷ Dentist는 치과의사이다. Dentists는 사람들이 치아를 깨끗하게 유지하는 것을 돕고 치아 및 잇몸질환을 치료한다. 사람들이 충치나 치통이 있을 때 Dentists를 방문한다.

❸ Pediatrician은 소아과의사이다. Pediatricians은 어린아이들을 치료하고 많은 종류의 질병을 치료해 줄 수 있다. 아이들이 독감이나 복통을 느끼면 Pediatricians을 찾는다.

❹ Oncologist는 종양학자/암연구자이다. Oncologists는 많은 종류의 암을 진단하고 치료하는 것을 돕는다. 사람들이 혹시 암에 걸리지 않았을까라고 걱정하면 Oncologists에 찾아간다.

C. Reading Practice 3

안녕하세요, 학생여러분. 오늘 우리는 의사들의 종류에 대해서 배울거예요. 여러분들 대부분이 아마도 이미 의사의 종류가 하나 이상이라는 것을 알고 있을 거예요. 그런데, 얼마나 많은 의사의 종류가 있는지를 알면 여러분들은 놀랄울 거예요. 총합해서, 60 이상의 다양한 의사들이 있고, 각각의 의사들은 몇몇 분야에 대해서 전공으로 하고 있어요. 자, 이제 각각의 종류에 대해 알아봅시다. 가장 흔한 의사는 바로 일반의라고 해요. 일반의들은 가정의이기도해요. 그들은 환자들이 보는 첫 번째 의사이고, 일반적인 질병을 다룹니다. 또 다른 종류에는 심장병 전문의가 있어요. 심장병 전문의들은 심장에 관련된 의사예요. 그들은 심장관련 질환들과 심장마비를 일으켰던 사람들을 치료합니다. 의사의 세 번째 종류에는 신경과 전문의가 있어요. 신경과 전문의들은 신경체계에 관련된 문제들을 다룹니다. 그 문제들은 두뇌, 척수, 신경, 또는 근육과 관련된 것들을 포함해요. 제가 오늘 말하려는 마지막 종류의 의사는 산부인과 전문의예요. 그들은 임신과 관련된 의사들이에요. 산부인과 전문의들은 임신한 여성들을 치료해줘요.

D. Reading Practice 4

Jeff **J**   Mom **M**

J 엄마! 더 많이 있어요! 매일 더 많이 있어요!

M Jeff야, 진정하렴. 무슨 말 하는거니?

J 여드름이요, 엄마. 매일 매일 여드름이 더 생겨요. 엄만 더 이상 제 얼굴을 못 볼거예요.

M 오, 우습긴/바보 같은 소리 하지마. 네 얼굴 좋아 보여. 네 또래 아이들이 여드름이 있는 건 당연한 일이야.

J 아니에요. 제 친구들 아무도 이 만큼의 여드름이 없어요

M 좋아. 내가 봤을 땐, 이게 필요하다고 생각하지 않는데...
그런데 네가 정 원하면, 학교 마치고 의사선생님께 널 데려다 줄게.
좀 진정하겠니?

J 의사선생님이 제 여드름에 대해 뭘 해줄 수 있을까요?

M 음, 일반의사말고, 피부과전문의. 피부과전문의들은 피부에 관련된 의사들인데 네 여드름이 더 빨리 없어질 수 있도록 도와주는 약을 줄거야.

J 정말요? 완벽하네요.

M 좋아, Jeff. 오늘 오후 4시에 우리가 피부과 의사선생님께 갈 수 있도록 예약을 해놓을께. 괜찮겠니?

J 좋아요! 고마워요, 엄마!

M 좋아, 내가 학교에 데려다 줄 수 있게 준비를 좀 마무리하겠니?

J 네, 5분만 기다려 주세요.

5. Narrative

01. 나는 치과에 가기 싫어요.

나는 치과에 갈 시간이 되면 도망가고 숨어요.

나는 매일 이를 닦아요. 그러나 아직도 충치가 있어요.

3개월마다 나는 치과에 갑니다.

그 시간은 무섭고 고통스러워요. 나는 치과의사 선생님이 싫어요.

내가 치과의사 선생님을 미워하는 것은 그리 놀라운 일이 아니에요.

치과병원 약 냄새도 나고 조명도 너무 밝아요. 날카로운 도구가 보여요.

공기와 물을 쏘는 작은 호스가 있어요.

그것들은 내 입안으로 넣는데 마치 진공청소기 같아요.

마지막으로 치과선생님 그의 손가락에 기구를 들고 제 입으로 가져가요.

그는 나의 잇몸에 이상한 물건을 넣기 시작했어요. 난 아무 말도 할 수 없어요.

나는 큰 주사를 나의 입안에 넣는 그의 손을 낚아챘어요.

나는 거의 의자에서 뛰어나왔어요. 그는 하지 말라고 말했어요.

하지만 했어요. 그는 나에게 소리쳤어요.

"움직이지마"

"론, 네가 움직이면 더 위험스러울 뿐이야!"

"론, 너는 더욱 양치질이 필요해" 그 다음에 그는 조금의 거즈를 가져다 대었어요.

그는 출혈을 멈추게 했어요. 내 인생 최악의 경험이었어요.

오늘 엄마가 치과의사 선생님께서 새로운 것을 갖고 있다고 말했어요.

엄마는 그것들이 멋있어 보인다고 말했어요.

먼저 치과의사 선생님이 잇몸을 문질렀는데, 그것은 사탕 같은 맛이에요.

막대기 모양이였는데 많이 본 볼펜 같이 생겼어요.

그건 정말 가는 바늘이 있었어요.

"너는 느낌조차 못 느낄거야" 그는 말했어요.

"곧 입안이 마비가 될거야" "그런 다음 넌 아름다운 미소와 함께 집으로 돌아갈 거야"

지금 아무리 그 말이 맞다 해도 나는 아직도 치과의사선생님이 싫어요.

02. 치아 요정을 만나다.

어느 날 클레어가 학교에서 집으로 뛰어왔어요.

그녀는 그녀의 엄마에게 미소를 지었어요.

"오늘은 다르게 보이는데?" "무슨 일이야?" 엄마가 물었어요.

클레어가 웃으며 물었어요. "무언가 없어진 게 보이나요?"

"없어지다니? 너의 치아!" 그녀의 엄마는 말했어요.

그리고 그녀의 입을 가리켰어요.

클레어는 그녀의 엄마에게 빠진 치아를 보여주었어요.

엄마가 말하기를 "음, 곧 치아 요정이 올 것 같은 생각이 드는데"

클레어는 그날 밤 잠자리에 일찍 들었어요.

그녀는 베개 밑에 치아를 넣어 두었어요. 그녀는 하품을 하고 기지개를 폈어요.

그녀는 곧 그녀의 곰인형 테디와 함께 잠이 들었어요.

클레어는 아주 작은 요정의 꿈을 꾸었어요.

그녀는 클레어에게 날아와 춤을 춥니다.

클레어는 그녀에게 미소를 지으며 질문을 했어요.

"너는 빠진 치아를 모아서 어디에다 보관하니?"

요정은 춤을 멈추고 행복하게 대답을 했어요.

"나는 무지개의 반대쪽에 분홍색 구름 안에 보관을 하지"

"환상적이야!" 클레어는 소리쳤어요.

갑자기 밤에 무언가가 클레어를 보니 소리가 들렸어요.

그녀는 어둠 속에서 주위를 둘러 보았어요.

빛이 방을 가로 질러 깜빡였어요.

클레어는 겁에 질렸어요. 그녀는 이불 밑으로 숨었어요.

"그건 뭐야?" 클레어는 궁금했어요. 클레어가 이불 속에서 살짝 나왔어요.

그녀는 다시 빛을 보았어요.

그것은 방을 가로질러 날아갔어요. 그것은 그녀의 침실 방문으로 빠져갔어요.

"그 빛이 치아 요정일까?" 클레어는 그녀 자신에게 물었어요.

그녀는 침대에 누웠어요. 클레어는 그녀의 베개 밑에 뭔가 움직이는 걸 느꼈어요.

그녀는 베개 밑을 살짝 보았는데 그녀의 치아는 사라졌어요.

그 대신에 반짝이는 은색 동전이 있었어요.

그녀는 너무 흥분했어요. 그녀는 테디에게 물었어요.

"너는 뭔가를 보았어?" 테디는 아무 말도 못했어요.

그녀의 손에 동전이 있었어요. 클레어는 다시 잠이 들었어요.

아침에 클레어는 동전을 보았어요.

그녀는 이 모든게 꿈인지 아닌지 궁금했답니다.

03. 아써의 치아 -마크브라운-

마지막으로 아써가 마지막 느슨한 치아 이야기를 했다.

마침내 아써는 치아가 흔들리기 시작했어요.

그는 혀로 치아를 흔들거렸어요.

그는 손가락으로도 치아를 흔들었어요.

그는 하루 종일 치아를 흔들거렸어요.

어느 날 오후, 아써가 수학시간에 자신의 치아를 흔들거리는 동안, 그는 큰 비명소리를 들었어요.

프랜신이 갑자기 날뛰면서 치아가 빠졌다고 소리를 쳤어요.

여러분, 여러분 중에 치아가 빠진 사람들이 몇 명이죠? 마르코 선생님이 물었습니다. 아써를 제외한 모든 사람이 손을 들었습니다.

아써가 집에 왔을 때 그는 우유와 쿠키를 먹고 싶지 않았어요.

"아써, 무슨 문제라도 있는 거야?" 그의 어머니가 물었어요.

"나 혼자만이 유일하게 젖니를 가지고 있어" 그는 불평을 했어요.

"걱정마" 그의 누나 DW가 말했어요. "너도 모든 치아가 빠진다는 것을 알고 있을 것이고, 쏘라 할머니처럼 틀니를 할 수도 있어" 누나가 말했습니다.

아써는 아써를 위해 특별한 만찬을: 스테이크, 옥수수, 땅콩 등을 준비하는 아버지를 위해 납득을 시켰습니다.

"이토록 작은 젖니가 빠지는데 오랜동안 시간이 걸리는지 믿을 수가 없어요" 아빠가 말했어요.

다음 날, 머피는 빠진 젖니를 위한 항아리를 가지고 왔어요. "나는 각 하나에 2달러를 받을 수가 있어" 그녀가 보여주면서 말했어요. 치아 하나는 아빠, 하나는 엄마 "나는 은행에 저금을 해서 이자를 받을 수 있지. 나는 내가 저금한 돈의 두 배가 되기를 기다고 있어"

"난 아냐, 난 그 돈을 가지고 나를 위해서 쓸 뿐이야" 프랜신이 말했다.

오후에 학급친구들은 더러운 충치 아저씨라는 영화를 보았어요.

"4살에서 7살 사이에 모든 사람들은 젖니, 즉 유치가 탈락하기 시작합니다" 라고 해설자가 설명했습니다.

"아써만 빼구요" 프랜신이 소리쳤어요.

교실에 있는 모든 친구들이 웃었어요.

아써가 미끄러지듯이 주저앉았고, 그는 할 수 있는 한 최선을 다해 자신의 치아를 흔들었어요.

학교식당에서 프랜신이 새로운 놀이를 연습했어요.

"봐라! 내 치아를 꽉 다물고도 여전히 빨대를 가지고 음료를 마실 수 있어."

"그리고 물총처럼 물을 뿜을 수도 있어. 여러분! 물총대회를 위해 줄을 서봐. 아써만 빼고 모두 다" 그녀는 말했어요.

"젖니를 가지고 있는 어린 아가들은 물총 놀이를 할 수가 없어"

다음 날까지 아써는 흔들거리는 치아가 더 이상 빠지지 않을 것이라고 확신했어요.

그의 친구들이 도움을 주기로 했어요.

버스터는 아써의 점심으로 당근을 가져왔고.

수 엘렌은 아써의 치아가 빠진 것처럼 보이게 하기 위해 건포도를 넣을 수 있다는 것을 보여주었어요.

브레인은 특별한 기계를 발명했어요.

이것은 "치아 제거기" 라고 설명했어요.

"그냥 여기에 머리를 넣어"

빙키 반즈도 도움을 주고 싶었어요.

"나는 한방에 네 치아를 넉다운 시킬 수 있어"

그날 밤 아써가 욕실 거울 앞에서 많은 시간을 보냈어요.

그는 그 다음날 일찍 일어나서 또 다시 그의 치아를 흔들기 시작했어요.

"얼만큼 치아가 더 흔들렸는지 봐 주세요" 그는 부모님께 말했어요.

"그만해" 라고 어머니가 대답을 했습니다.

"전문가의 도움이 필요하겠어. 오늘 치과에 함 가보자꾸나"

"치과에 가는 것?" 프랜신이 말했다.

"이 녀석아. 내가 너에게 유감스럽다고 해야 하나?"

소지오 치과선생님의 치료를 받기 위해 기다리는 환자들이 있었어요.

"미안한데 환자들이 좀 밀려서 조금 기다려야 할 것 같아" 간호사 선생님이 말했어요. "앉아서 기다려라"

"똑똑한 아써야 책을 읽으면서 기다리자꾸나"

어머니가 말했어요.

마침내 아써의 차례가 되었어요.

"모든 환자들이 너처럼 기다리기를 잘 할 수 있기를 바랄뿐이야" 소지오 치과선생님께서 말했어요. "아써야. 지금 몇 살이니?"

"일곱살이요," 아써가 대답했어요.

"나는 8살 때 젖니가 빠졌어 모든 사람들은 빠지는 시기가 달라" 소지오 치과선생님이 그렇게 말했어요.

"정말요?" 아써가 되물었어요.

소지오 선생님은 아써의 흔들리는 젖니를 검진하였어요.

"좀 더 기다려봐. 치아가 곧 빠질거야" 선생님께서 설명해주셨어요.

아써는 쉬는 시간 학교로 왔습니다. "너 여전히 젖니가 있는 거야?" 프랜신에게 물었다.

"그럼 너는 이 게임을 할 수가 없어. 나는 치아 요정이고. 젖니가 빠진 사람만이 이 게임을 할 수가 있어"

"만약 네가 치아 요정이라면" 아써가 말했어요.

"나는 내 치아를 지키겠어, 그래... 기다릴 수 있어"

그는 소프트볼 게임을 시작했어요.

"나는 젖니가 빠진 사람을 잡을 수 있어" 프랜신은 말했어요.

그녀는 자신의 팔을 퍼덕거렸어요. "치아가 가장 많이 빠진 단 한 사람이 승리하는 것이야."

프랜신은 빙글빙글 돌면서 버스터를 터치했어요.

더 빨리 돌면서 수 알렌을 터치했어요.

그녀는 심지어 더 빠르게 돌며 미끄러져서 아써를 툭 쳤어요.

"미안해, 근데 아기들은 할 수 없다고 내가 말했잖아." 프랜신이 말했어요.

아써는 안경을 집어 들면서 "괜찮아"라고 말했어요.

"아마도 네가 나한테 해준 것 중에 가장 좋은 일을 해준 것 같아."

"무슨 말이니?" 프랜신이 물었어요.

아써는 그저 미소만 지었어요.

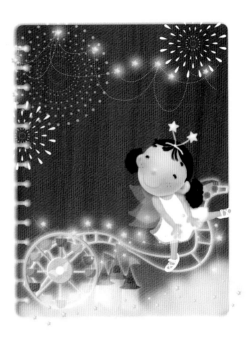

Answer

1. Vocabulary

Exercise 1 (병원에서 사용하는 단어 I)

Ⓐ 1.2.3 생략

Ⓑ 빈칸에 들어갈 알맞은 것을 〈보기〉에서 고르시오.

  1. bruise 2. fatal 3. unconscious 4. choked

Ⓒ 밑줄 친 부분과 뜻이 가장 가까운 것을 고르시오.

  1. (d) 2. (e) 3. (e) 4. (b)

Exercise 2 (병원에서 사용하는 단어 II)

Ⓐ 1.2.3 생략

Ⓑ 빈칸에 들어갈 알맞은 것을 〈보기〉에서 고르시오.

  1. paralyzed 2. prescription 3. organs 4. cured

Ⓒ 밑줄 친 부분과 뜻이 가장 가까운 것을 고르시오.

  1. (e) 2. (b) 3. (c) 4. (a)

Exercise 3 (질병 및 증상을 나타내는 단어)

Ⓐ 1.2.3 생략

Ⓑ 빈칸에 들어갈 알맞은 것을 〈보기〉에서 고르시오.

  1. leukemia 2. arthritis 3. diabetes 4. asthma

Ⓒ 밑줄 친 부분과 뜻이 가장 가까운 것을 고르시오.

  1. (d) 2. (e) 3. (b) 4. (a)

Exercise 4 (기타 건강관련 단어)

Ⓐ 1.2.3 생략

Ⓑ 빈칸에 들어갈 알맞은 것을 〈보기〉에서 고르시오.

  1. cramps 2. numb 3. limped 4. deaf

Ⓒ 밑줄 친 부분과 뜻이 가장 가까운 것을 고르시오.

  1. (b) 2. (b) 3. (c) 4. (e)

Ⓓ Fill in the blanks with the correct word or expression from the list below.

  1. runny, sneeze 2. allergic 3. bruise

4. sore throat 5. chills 6. diarrhea 7. faint

8. itchy 9. fever 10. scratch 11. swollen

12. contagious 13. rash 14. dizzy, hangover

15. vomit, nauseated

치과 전문용어와 환자 눈높이의 표현법

dental terminology	dental expression for patient	korean meaning
abscess	infection in a tooth	농양
analgesic	pain medicine / pain killers	진통제
anterior tooth	front tooth	전치
buccal	cheek side of the tooth	협측의
calculus	calcium deposits on teeth	치석
carcinoma	cancer	암
cariogenic	decay producing	우식을 유발하는
carious lesion	cavity / tooth decay	우식병소
composite resin	tooth-colored filling	복합레진
crown	cap	금관
curette	instrument for cleaning teeth	큐렛
cusp	top of the tooth	교두
dental caries	cavity/tooth decay	치아우식증
dentifrice	toothpaste	치약
dentition	teeth	치열
endodontic therapy	root canal treatment	근관치료
first molar	six-year molar	제1대구치
fixed prosthesis	bridge	가공의치
gingivitis	early gum disease	치은염
halitosis	bad breath	구취
impression	mold of the teeth	인상
incisor	front teeth	절치
injection	shot	주사
lingual	tongue side of the tooth	설측

dental terminology	dental expression for patient	korean meaning
malocclusion	misalignment of the teeth	부정교합
mandible	lower jaw	하악골
maxilla	upper jaw	상악골
molar	back tooth	대구치
occlusal surface	chewing surface	교합면
oral	mouth	구강
oral prophylaxis	teeth cleaning	치면세마
orthodonic treatment	braces	교정치료
pedodontist	children's dentist	소아치과 전문의
periodontal disease	gum disease	치주질환
periodontal surgery	gum surgery	치주외과
periodontal tissue	gums	치주조직
periodontist	gum disease specialist	치주과 전문의
pit and fissures	grooves in teeth	소아열구
pit and fissure sealant	sealant	전색제
plaque	bacteria on teeth	치면세균막
posterior tooth	back tooth	구치
primary dentition	baby teeth	유치
radiograph	X-ray	방사선사진
removable prosthesis	removable denture	가철성 보철물
restoration	filling	수복
root planing	deep cleaning	치근활택술
saliva	spit	침
scaler	instrument for clening teeth	치은연하의
scaling	removal of calculus and deposits	치석제거
subgingival	below the gum line	치석제거기
supernumeray tooth	extra tooth	과잉치
temporomandibular joint	jaw joint	악관절
third molar	wisdom tooth	제3대구치

Exercise 5 (치과 영어 표현법)

Ⓐ Odd one out

1. thumb – It is not part of leg or feet.
2. knee – It is not part of arm.
3. hip – It is not.
4. calf – It is not part of head.
5. tongue – It is not part of hand.
6. knuckle – It is not part of eye.
7. nail – It is not part of hair.
8. shoulder – It is not part of leg.
9. neck – It is not an internal organ.
10. cheek – It is not part of mouth.

Ⓑ Name the body part.

1. nose   2. teeth   3. brain   4. beard   5. fingers
6. throat   7. moustache   8. neck   9. elbow
10. wrist   11. ankle   12. knee
13. tongue(mouth, teeth, lips)   14. chest

3. Reading Comprehension

Exercise 6

Ⓐ What is the secret word?

Brush / plague / apple / floss / cavity / dentist
tooth / smiles / The secret word is sealant

Exercise 7

Ⓐ Fill-in the blank game.

1. sweet, nutritious 2. fluoride, teeth
3. decay, smiling 4. dentist brush, floss
5. visited, sealants, molars 6. plaque, snacks
7. happy

06 I feel terrible

terrible, stomachache, headache, pharmacy, medicine.

① Vocabulary preview
   1. (a) 2. (b) 3. (b)

② Key expressions
   1. (b) 2. (c) 3. (a)

③ Dialogue
   1. (c) 2. (b) 3. (f) 4. (a) 5. (d)

④ Questions Answers
   생략

⑤ On your Own
   생략

⑥ Quiz
   A. 1. medicine 2. stomachache
      3. Pharmacy 4. headache
   B. 1. (b) 2. (a)
   C. 1. I don't feel very good.
      2. I feel terrible.
      3. My head feels hot.
      4. Let me feel your forehead.
      5. I guess you're right.
      6. I'll get some medicine at the pharmacy.
      7. Take this medicine.
      8. You'd better stay in today.
      9. I have a headache.
      10. Do I need some medicine.

07 Visiting the Doctor

   A. 1. medicine 2. bandage 3. sneeze 4. shot
   B. 1. checks 2. coughs 3. fever 4. stomachache
   C. ⓐ medicine ⓑ sneeze / cough ⓒ bandage
      ⓓ stomachache

① Reading
   A. 1. (d) 2. (b)
   B. 1. (c) 2. (b)
   C. (d)

② Quiz
   A. (c), (a), (b)
   B. 1. (c) 2. (a) 3. (d)
   C. (c) → (a) → (d) → (b)

08. Health and Safety

① Warming up
   A. 1. How are you feeling today?
      2. She is going to take your temperature.
      3. You should go to bed and rest.
      4. My sister has an ankle sprained.
   B. 1. Yes, they were.
      2. ex) I do exercise everyday.
      3. ex) I go to the gym to exercise every morning.
      4. ex) I sleep about eight hours.

② Answer the fitness quiz
   A. 생략
   B. 1. (a) T (b) F (C) T (d) F
      2. ex) Mandy should drink more water.
            Mandy should take a rest.
            Mandy should go to bed early.
      3. 생략

09. What do you know about healthcare?

② Guess What
   1. injection 2. bandage 3. bleeding 4. check-up
   5. EKG 6. measles 7. painkillers 8. dental floss

④ Reading

A. 1. (b)

2. To ease the pain

B. 1. (b)

2. (a) 4   (b) 1   (c) 2   (d) 3

C. 1. (d)

2. (a) T   (b) T   (c) T

3. On your own

Skin rash / runny nose / stomachache / cough / feeling tired / eating sleeping problem

D. 1. (b)   2. (a)

E. 1. (b)

2. They take foundation course such as a chemistry, biology and physiology.

3. (a) T (b) F (c) F

4. Nursing degree: a four- year program.

　* In the first two years: take foundation course

　* In the last two years: work in a hospital with patients work under the supervision of doctors.

　* In the final year: give patients injection and assist doctors.

F. 1. (b)

2. cavities, gum disease, cancer

3. (a) T (b) F (c) F

4. Every day regularly

　- brush after every meal

　- use dental floss

Dental check-up

　- visit your dentist twice a year

　+ can detect cavities ? easy to fix

　+ can detect gum disease ? treat it early

　+ can detect cancer

　　ex. oral cancer

4. Dialogue

01 Dental English

⑥ Dialogue 6

A. (b) B. (a)   C. (a) D. (c) E. (a)

02. Which doctor should I go to?

① Let's get started

A. Warm-up questions

1. There are dentist, pediatrician, heart doctors.

2. When I am sick, I go to a pediatrician, who is a special doctor for children.

B. 1. diagnose 2. zit 3. pediatrician 4. treat

5. neurologist 6. optometrist 7. disease

8. cardiologist

② Let's read

A. 1. (b) 2. (b) 3. (d)

B. Reading practice 2

1. Dermatologist

(a) Definition: skin doctor

(b) Job description: help people who have skin problems and treat different skin disease.

(c) Reasons to visit: If they get burned or have problems with zits.

2. Dentist

(a) Definition: tooth doctor

(b) Job description: help people keep their teeth clean and treat tooth and gum disease.

(c) Reasons to visit: If they have cavities or a toothache.

3. Pediatrician

(a) Definition: Special doctor for children.

(b) Job description: help young children and treat lots of different illness.

(c) Reasons to visit: If they have the flu or a stomachache.

4. Oncologist

(a) Definition: Cancer doctor

(b) Job description: help diagnosis and treat different types of cancer.

(c) Reasons to visit: If they are worried, they might have cancer.

C. Reading practice 3

1. General practitioners: family doctors.

They treat general sickness.

2. Cardiologists: heart doctors.

They treat hear disease.

3. Neurologists: nervous system doctors.

They treat problems of the nervous system.

4. Obstetricians: pregnancy doctors.

They treat women who are pregnant.

D. Reading practice 4

Task 1   ✓ Which doctor to go to

Task 2   1. (a) 2. (c) 3. (c)

③ Let's talk

1. 생략

④ Read and number

8 – 1 – 7 – 4 – 10 – 11 – 5 – 6 – 3 – 9 – 2

⑤ Based Lessons

A. 1. (d) 2. (g) 3. (m) 4. (i) 5. (k) 6. (n) 7. (l) 8. (f)

9. (c) 10. (a) 11. (e) 12. (h) 13. (b) 14. (j)

B. 1. (d) 2. (f) 3. (h) 4. (g) 5. (i) 6. (j) 7. (a) 8. (c)

9. (b) 10. (d)

5. Narrative

Story 1. I hate going to the Dentist

VOCABULARY BUILD UP

Ⓐ Match the words to the correct definitions.

1. (i) 2. (d) 3. (b) 4. (g) 5. (f)

6. (e) 7. (h) 8. (c) 9. (a)

Ⓑ Choose the best words to fill in the blankets.

1. (b) 2. (b) 3. (a) 4. (b) 5. (b)

COMPREHENSION CHECK UP

Ⓐ Check true or false.

1. F 2. F

Ⓑ Choose the best answers.

1. (a) 2. (b) 3. (c) 4. (c)

Story 2. Meeting the Tooth Fairy

VOCABULARY BUILD UP

Ⓐ Match the words to the correct definitions.

1. (f) 2. (g) 3. (h) 4. (a) 5. (e) 6. (d) 7. (b) 8. (c)

Ⓑ Choose the best words to fill in the blankets.

1. (d) 2. (d) 3. (b) 4. (c) 5. (d)

COMPREHENSION CHECK UP

Ⓐ Check true or false.

1. T 2. F

Ⓑ Choose the best answers.

1. (b) 2. (a) 3. (d) 4. (d)